THE THINKING BODY

Clemence Bettany was born and educated in Australia and trained as a ballet dancer, making her debut in Paris with Roland Petit's Les Ballets de Paris. Injury, marriage and motherhood cut short her career and she now divides her time between teaching, researching and lecturing about movement and skeletal alignment techniques. She is an active member of the Campaign for the Advancement of State Education (CASE).

Christopher Poulton was born and educated in New Zealand, where he studied photography. He travelled extensively throughout Australia before arriving in England where he continued his studies at the City and Guilds Art School, specializing in sculpture. He now teaches sculpture, and is currently working towards a major exhibition of his own work.

THE THINKING BODY

Clemence Bettany

Illustrated by Christopher Poulton

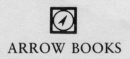

ARROW BOOKS

For Jane Clayton

Arrow Books Limited
62–65 Chandos Place, London WC2N 4NW

An imprint of Century Hutchinson Limited

London Melbourne Sydney Auckland
Johannesburg and agencies throughout
the world

First published 1989

Phototypeset by Input Typesetting Ltd, London
Printed and bound in Great Britain by
The Guernsey Press Co Ltd,
Guernsey, Channel Islands

ISBN 0 09 955080 6

Contents

The chapter titles are from Cole Porter lyrics:
Chapter 1 – from the song 'I worship you'
  (*Fifty Million Frenchmen*, 1929)
Chapter 2 – from the song of the same title
  (*Born to Dance*, 1936)
Chapter 3 – from the song of the same title
  (*Star Dust*, 1931)
Chapter 4 – from the song 'At long last love'
  (*You Never Know*, 1938)

ACKNOWLEDGMENTS

There are many people I owe — not just for the passing on of their knowledge but for their support and encouragement.

I would like to thank the late Leon Kellaway and Kathleen Gorham who instilled in a young girl a belief in the expressive qualities of the body, as well as the late Audrey de Vos, one of the first dance teachers to realize that the body was governed by anatomical principles. For my own subsequent initiation into those principles, I have to thank a remarkable teacher and therapist, Jean Gibson.

Often the chance remark, a name dropped into the conversation, pulls you unknowingly in the right direction. Such was the case when, in the course of a lecture, Kedzie Penfield mentioned the name of Lulu Sweigard and her work at the Juilliard School. Through Sweigard, I made the acquaintance of a book written by Mabel Elsworth Todd, whose title I have unashamedly borrowed, there being no better description, as she so unerringly knew.

My thanks also to Bonnie Bainbridge Cohen, to Heather Williams and Marion Gough, and to Scott Clark who confirmed my view that mental sweat achieved more than the damp variety. Finally, I am immensely grateful to my friends and students, in particular Margo Cooper, Sylvia Mingay and Judith Burnley, as well as my mother-in-law and my mother, without whose support during the writing of this book the household would surely have foundered.

Clemence Bettany
London, 1988

CHAPTER 1

'Back in the days when Greece was mighty'

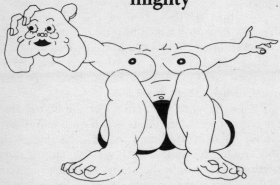

'To the neurologist . . . it is readily apparent that the sole product of brain function is motor co-ordination. To repeat: the entire output of our thinking machine consists of nothing but patterns of motor co-ordination.

'It follows that the principal function of the nervous system is the co-ordinated innervation of the musculature. Its fundamental anatomical plan and working principles are understandable only on these terms.'

Roger Sperry, Nobel Prize for Physiology & Medicine, 1981.[1]

From the beginning of time, men have endeavoured to explain themselves to themselves, trying to make sense of the known and unknown. What could be seen and touched like a body was explicably human. What could not, like the mind, was by definition mysterious. It was inconceivable that the repulsive contents of a skull could account for a Socrates or a Plato or an Aristotle. The mind had to be a gift from the gods; there was no other acceptable explanation. Pythagoras, the vegetarian of the isosceles triangle, believed that the human soul[2] came from God and needed to be kept away from contamination (the Greeks having no word for sin) by the body.

Later, Plato too put the case for divine creation. Gods, upon
instruction from a creator God, 'copied the shape of the universe
and fastened the two divine orbits of the soul into a spherical
body, which we now call the head, the divinest part of us which
controls all the rest . . . then put together the body as a whole
to serve the head.'[3]

Elaborating on this, he then divided the whole into three
souls: one divine – Reason – which he situated in the head, and
two mortal – Emotion and Appetite. So that these mortal souls
would not pollute 'the divine element', they were located in the
body 'with the neck as a kind of isthmus and boundary between
head and breast to keep them apart.'[4]

Surprisingly enough, when the authors of the first chapter of
Genesis got together to put their ideas down on paper, they held
a different view: 'God created man in his own image, in the
image of God created he him.' There was no suggestion that
man was anything but whole. Later, in the New Testament,
when John talked about the coming of Jesus, he wrote: 'And
the Word was made flesh . . .' There was no suggestion here
either that 'flesh' was other than a fit substance for the Son of
God.

'Truth,' Bacon argued, 'is not the daughter of authority but
of time.'[5] Regrettably truth rarely survives a second telling, let
alone the passage of time. When St Augustine made his appear-
ance in the fifth century AD, the association of the flesh with
the devil was more familiar than with Jesus Christ. St Augustine
was forced to defend the use of the word 'flesh' by pointing out
that it was merely another way of saying that the Word had
been made human.

To his credit, St Augustine pointed out that 'sin came from
the soul, and not the flesh.'[6] A point which unfortunately didn't
receive the attention it deserved. Carnality, originally just
another word for corporeality, was to be forever lewd.

The change that took place in the intention of the word 'flesh'
can be traced in the dictionary. Before the middle of the twelfth
century, it was used, in a biblical sense, to mean 'the physical
frame of man: the body'. By the middle of the fifteenth, its
significance had been crucially altered to mean 'the depraved

nature of man in its conflict with the promptings of the Spirit'.

Today's child, if his or her parents are Anglican, will encounter the word 'lust' in church before he or she has any notion of its meaning. The Catechism asks that the child renounce not only the 'devil and all his works, the pomps and vanity of this wicked world' but 'all the sinful lusts of the flesh' as well.

The separation of mind and body proposed by the Hellenic Greeks was taken on board by the early Christian Church, despite St Augustine's refutation of Plato 'in ascribing sin unto the nature of the flesh'.[7]

Most of us assume that what was believed in the fifth century BC or AD is hardly relevant in the twentieth, except as history. Yet underneath today's attitudes there flows this river of yesterday's beliefs carrying us unknowingly along. Once the body had sin on a name tag around its neck, it was deserving of punishment. Though the more extreme forms of physical punishment have now been outlawed by most Western nations (we no longer gouge out eyes or cut off ears, castrate or practise flagellation), belief in the efficacy of physical punishment is still widely held whether it be only a smack, a slap; or a 'good thrashing'. The use of the cane in British state schools has only recently been banned, and is still permissible in independent schools.

We may go to an exercise class with the best of intentions to improve our health, but if it didn't bring us out in a sweat we wouldn't go back. Mortifying the flesh lives on under the name of aerobics – physical jerks set to different music. The exultation felt after 'the burn' can be likened to that felt by the medieval flagellant.

Separation of mind and body is immortalised in phrases like 'mental arithmetic', 'physical exercise'; institutionalised in school time-tables – a direct legacy of an age in which physical exercise was taught alongside reading and writing and music in the Gymnasia. Though a healthy mind in a healthy body was one Plato endorsed: – '. . . anyone engaged on mathematics or any other strenuous intellectual pursuit should also exercise his body and take part in physical training; while the man who devotes his attention to physical fitness should correspondingly take mental exercise and have cultural and intellectual interests'[8] – there was never any question of equality between the two. Physical training was largely intended not only to develop prowess but to inculcate qualities of stamina and courage; after all, the Greek city-states were on an almost continuous war footing.

Reporters of modern-day sporting events litter their copy with fighting analogies. Meetings are described as 'confrontations' whether they be between man and stopwatch, man and man, team and team, nation and nation; winners frequently scale 'new heights of heroism' and the result is often hailed as 'a victory'. Sport has never been a simple celebration of body skill – rather a means to winning a more glorious end.

As succeeding generations rediscovered the Greek philosophers, the worlds of mind and body were driven further apart. Though the Renaissance brought them briefly together, it was not long before Descartes came along with a pair of scissors, cutting off the mind once more to spite the body, with his famous one-liner: 'I think therefore I am.'

At first reading, Descartes appeared to believe in the integrity of the brain and body: '. . . I am not only lodged in my body, like a pilot in his ship, but, besides, that I am joined to it very closely and indeed so compounded and intermingled with my body, that I form, as it were, a single whole with it.'[9]

But the brain was not the mind: 'And although perhaps (or rather as I shall shortly say, certainly,) I have a body to which I am very closely united, nevertheless, because, on the one hand, I have a clear and distinct idea of myself in so far as I am only a thinking and unextended thing but which does not think, it is certain that I, that is to say my mind, by which I am what I am, is entirely and truly distinct from my body, and may exist without.'[10] Perhaps he should have stuck to the one-liners.

Through the use of his beloved analytical geometry, Descartes believed that the world could be worked out on a piece of paper; there was no limit to what the mind could do. The scientific revolution which followed the philosopher from La Haye raised the prestige of the mind at the expense of the body, and the industrial revolution went a stage further in preferring the machine to the man. Though the body had been on the skids for some time, now it reached rock bottom. The simulation of body skills by twentieth-century machines is so much a part of our lives that it has never occurred to us to think of what we may have lost instead of what we have gained.

It comes as a shock then to discover that there may be no evidence for the assumption of superiority of mind over body, that there may be no qualitative difference between mental and physical activity, that the brain cells destined for weighty intellectual matters may be no different to those detailed for gross physical work, that the dressing room had after all, no star pinned to the door.

'It is not the quality of the sensory nerve impulses that determines their conscious properties but rather the different areas of the brain into which they discharge. The difference between one mental state and another is accordingly believed to depend upon variance in the timing and distribution of nerve excitations, not upon differences in quality among the individual impulses' (Roger Sperry).[11]

You may well wonder why you haven't come across this information before, why it hasn't been more widely circulated and become common knowledge.

Contrary to what we like to think, our sensory apparatus is programmed to keep the blinkers on, only cautiously selecting from the mass of information with which it is bombarded.[12] The first reaction of the foetus to an external stimulus is not a turning toward but a turning away. Biological growth has been genetically programmed, presumably out of necessity, seeing how innately conservative we are.

Unfortunately, there appears to be no cultural programming – old ideas go on being recycled indefinitely by those who desire to keep the heirlooms in the family. According to Arthur Koestler, 'The inertia of the human mind and its resistance to innovation are most clearly demonstrated not, as one might expect, by the ignorant mass – which is easily swayed once its imagination is caught – but by professionals with a vested interest in tradition and in the monopoly of learning. Innovation is a twofold threat to academic mediocrities; it endangers their oracular authority, and it evokes the deeper fear that their whole, laboriously constructed intellectual edifice might collapse.'[13]

The past is the standard by which we judge the new, whether it be a car or an idea. But whereas with a car, it is the proven ability to do the job that influences us to buy another of the same make, with an idea there is no such rationale. On the contrary, it is the 'oracular' nature of the handing down that influences, the endorsements accompanying the message that give it credence, the sweet sales pitch that convinces. If we were indeed rational (as we like to think we are), we would see what a bad track record dualism has and refrain from pouring more good money after bad.

No one looking at us today – for the most part, awkward, ill co-ordinated, graceless, clumsy – would think that we possess the effortless skills of the animal. Only when we watch a great dancer or superb athlete do we catch a glimpse of what might have been. For most of us, the integration which distinguishes the great dancer, the athlete, the animal, is lacking.

Koestler wrote in *The Sleepwalkers*: '. . . a diseased state of organism, a society, or culture, is characterized by a weakening of the integrative controls, and the tendency of its parts to behave in an independent and self-assertive manner, ignoring the superior interest of the whole, or trying to impose their own laws on it. Such states of imbalance may be caused either by the weakening of the co-ordinating powers of the whole through growth beyond a critical limit, senescence, and so forth; or by excessive stimulation of an organ or part; or its cutting off from communication with the integrative centre.'[14]

What we think about our bodies is largely a matter of what we have been taught to think about them, and we appear to have been taught very little except that they are inferior. The inside of a vacuum cleaner, a car, an electric plug are all more familiar to us than our own bodies. If we were asked to draw a picture of them, we could be certain only of the outline. We may be taught the mechanics of sex and reproduction at school (before we have any coherent view of the whole body) but it is only in the fourth year of state secondary school that human biology makes its debut as a subject. Even then, it is often underrated in comparison to biology and offered as a suitable subject for the less able child. Despite our apparent sophistication in this post-permissive age, our attitudes to the body remain distinctly ambivalent.

The separation of mind and body might have seemed logical enough in Plato's time; without modern technology, how could he have known that the division was not as he imagined it? Today, with all our knowledge, we still ascribe different spheres of action for brain and body; we still reward the mind and abuse the body. Yet we know that the brain and the spinal cord which make up the central nervous system grow from the same neural tube, develop from the same nervous tissue; that the canal carrying cerebro-spinal fluid flows continuously from tail to brain; and that the ascending and descending fibres inside the cord pass messages from one spinal level to another, as well as to and from the brain. The mental process that results in a step is similar to that which results in a thought; the level of cerebration is determined by the complexity of either move or thought.

When we talk about the brain, we not only think of it as distinct from the rest of the central nervous system but as being functionally distinct as well – as being a single homogenous unit primarily devoted to thinking.[15]

But evolution has bequeathed us not one but many neural systems (of which the cerebral cortex is but the latest in evolutionary terms) and linked them in a complex pattern of pathways. Playing a sport, like playing an instrument, requires not just mute obedience of the body to the commands of the motor cortex but the integrated activity of the whole cortex.[16]

For over a century, it was generally agreed that though the two hemispheres of the brain were anatomically symmetrical, they were asymmetrical in function i.e. the left was concerned with language, the right with spatial functions. Naturally enough, given the cultural ethos, the left hemisphere was assumed to be the dominant one. As the right side of the body is largely controlled by the left hemisphere and vice versa, it was

thought that the right hand owed its superiority to the dominance of the left hemisphere.

It looked very much as if the superiority of mind over body
was a projection of the relationship between the two hemispheres. When in the 1960's, Roger Sperry's work on human
split-brain research revealed that when the central connection
between the two hemispheres, the corpus callosum, was cut (as
in cases of severe epilepsy) the right hemisphere was unable
to name recognisable objects, the case for cerebral dominance
appeared to have been won.

'When the brain is dissected,' Sperry wrote, 'we see two
separate "selves" – essentially a divided organism with its own
memories and its own will – competing for control over the
organism.'[17] In his James Arthur Lecture in 1964, Sperry went
a stage further: 'Evolution, of course, has made notable errors
in the past and one suspects that in the elaboration of the higher
brain centres evolutionary progress is more encumbered than
aided by the bilateralized scheme . . .'

Yet there was other evidence, exceptions to the rule, which,
though didn't contradict the idea of a left hemisphere concerned
with language and a right with spatial matters, suggested a
different interpretation.

Up to the age of four, children showed less hemispheric differentiation as far as language was concerned;[18] damage to one
hemisphere at an early age was offset by the other taking over.
Women's brains showed less differentiation than men's and were
less disadvantaged by damage to a hemisphere. Left-handed
individuals were found to have 'a more nearly equal bilateral
representation' with 'more diffuseness of language mechanisms
with the hemisphere contralateral to the dominant hand.'[19]

From these examples and many others, it was seen that
cerebral dominance, far from being a simple matter of one
hemisphere lauding it over the other, varied, not only from
function to function but also from person to person, age to age,
male to female.

As we approach the final decade of this century, it has become
clear that talk of dominant and non-dominant hemispheres is
no longer valid.[20]. Asymmetry is more than skin deep, it is built

into the structure of the brain and can be seen in the foetus as early as the 10th gestational week.[21] Though the classical neurological contention, that the left hemisphere is responsible for learning and using language, holds, it no longer follows that all components of speech are localised on the left or that all spatial components are localised on the right.[22] Individual zones of the cortex may be components of different systems, taking part in different functions. Though some cells only respond to certain stimuli, others are multi-sensory, responding to many different stimuli in different parts of the body. Movement like language is formed by participation between different neural systems. What Sperry suspected to be an evolutionary mistake might, even yet, turn out to be the partnership of the century, if not this one's then certainly the next.

Being born with a silver spoon in our mouths, so to speak, is unhappily no advantage to us while we are growing up. As babies, we are picked up by well-meaning parents who bring us what we want rather than let us inch our way towards it. They put us in baby-walkers to encourage us to walk as if they doubted we would take the plunge if left on our own. As our homes are full of objects both dangerous and precious, we are confined in play-pens or hemmed in to keep us on the spot. Outside, the grass in the park is covered with dog-shit and most playgrounds are coated with asphalt, so we are strapped safely in our baby buggies. Every day is accompanied by 'sit down', 'keep still', thwarting our efforts to practise. Once we are taken out of the nursery, we are expected to sit down for much of the day; music may feature in the state primary school curriculum, but not dance, and sport and PE receive no serious attention in the majority of state schools. At no time is recognition given to the fact that, as Roger Sperry says, 'Mental activity develops out of, and in reference to, overt action.'[23]

By the time we come of age, we have amassed a collection of postural malapropisms which are as inefficient as they are disruptive. By the time we enter middle age, we are likely to be in serious trouble. The way we habitually use the right hand for everything from reaching the jar on the shelf to picking up the baby, carrying the suitcase or shaking hands; the way we always

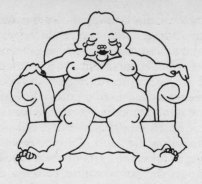

cross our legs, slump back in a chair, slouch at the bus stop, tense our shoulders, frown as we concentrate – leaves marks which become tramlines. Admittedly, there is little we can do while we are growing up, except press for more enlightened parents and a more enlightened educational system. But if our old age is not to be just a time of reckoning, we need to set about putting things right beforehand.

Putting things right means, first of all, getting to know your body. It is the most valuable piece of equipment you will ever own and, to use Descartes' famous analogy between man and clock, you don't shake a valuable timepiece in the hope that it will go better. If a machine is not performing well, you don't make it work harder. Unless the basic structure of the body is balanced, a dose of exercise is more likely to damage than cure. And you can only balance your body if you know something about its anatomy.

Getting to know yourself is not a question of being able to name names, it is, above all, being able to translate a diagram on the page into your own body, sensing not only with the eyes but with the fingers, touching what is palpable, using the imagination when it is not. It is a 'knowing' in the fullest sense of the word.

As you get to know how the parts fit together, how the delicate balance of bone on bone is maintained by ligaments, learn to recognise the work of different groups of muscles, your body will begin to translate that information into action by adjusting the slouch, the slump, the strain; de-stabilising old habits and substituting new ones. Normally, much of this adjusting will take place below the level of consciousness, but you can quicken the process by the use of self-awareness – in the manner of the man in the television studio who holds up a card telling you when to laugh or applaud, except in this case, the card shows you what you should be doing: the way the thigh bone fits into the hip socket, the curves of the spine, the position of the head on the neck, the placement of a muscle. But to be able to do this, your visualisation needs to be accurate and detailed – you need to have done your homework. A fuzzy image will produce an equally fuzzy response; an inaccurate image, the wrong response.

One of the tricks of the trade, used by professionals, is mental practice: the rehearsing of a move or a sequence of moves without lifting so much as a finger. To be successful, and it can be very successful in re-educating the body, you must take care not to skimp on the details and visualise every inch of the movement. It has the added advantage in that you need no rehearsal room; you can practise while you're on a train, lying in bed, feeding the baby, stuck in a traffic jam, waiting for a telephone call or sitting on the lav.

What you are doing is refining the concept of the movement, drawing up a better, more detailed plan for the brain to program. Whether it be the fingering for a tricky bar in a Beethoven Sonata, a forehand smash or sitting down, you can mentally prepare for it and rehearse it without getting out of the chair.

What you must not do is confuse or combine the two operations – the preparation and the performance – otherwise self-awareness will very quickly turn to self-consciousness. The patterning of muscular response is far too fast and intricate to be plotted consciously. The self who watches is like the good director, and a good director would never dream of acting out the performer's role.

'The process of evolution may be described as differentiation of structure and integration of function. The more differentiated and specialized the parts, the more elaborate coordination is needed to create a well-balanced whole. The ultimate criterion of the value of a functional whole is the degree of its internal harmony or integratedness, whether the "functional whole" is a biological species or a civilization or an individual.' (Arthur Koestler)[24]

You may well say to yourself that all you want is a body that works well, that is shapely as well as fit, but the human body is neither simple nor easy to comprehend. Functioning on just a few units of brain power – or on only the primitive reflexes of the brain – when you have the whole powerful battery at your disposal, is as absurd as someone driving a Rolls Royce in second gear with the hand-brake on.

The integration of the body depends on the mind. My body is as much an expression of my thought as is this sentence. And so is yours.

CHAPTER 2
'I've got you under my skin'

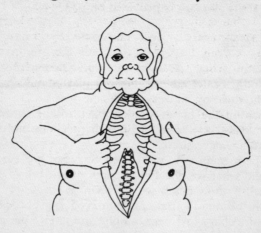

All movement is a combination of nerves, muscles and bones. Though by nature I am a holist, in this instance I propose to take the body apart and look at each part in turn before explaining how they work together.

Much of our physical efficiency depends on the alignment of the bones of the skeleton – an alignment calling for exactness, which, if we were machines, would not present a problem; precision would be ours to keep, if only for the guarantee period. But, because we are who we are – under siege from work, stress, habit – fixed precision escapes us.

Alignment of the human body, unlike that of the machine, is never constant; it is easily put out and needs frequent adjustment.

Obviously, bones by themselves cannot align the body. They are only part of a complex system of ligaments, tendons, muscles and nerves, which underpin, brace, bandage and joint the structure, breathing life into it. But without a knowledge of the framework, how can one understand the whole?

What follows is not a comprehensive tabling of every bone of the body, but a look at those crucial to the balancing of the body. The exercises set out are exercises in awareness and have little value other than to help you identify bones and joints.

Where possible, I have substituted popular names for medical terms. A short glossary is provided on page (100).

The skeleton

The skeleton is not a piece of sculpture. Bones (there are 206 of them in the body) are not metal or plaster and needing to be bent or moulded by an outside agency.

Cells within the bones not only see to the formation and growth but also to the repair and remodelling that stress and injury and age necessitate.

Their performance is influenced by what we eat, how we behave and what we do. The strength of our bones is partially determined by how much we use them.

After the Gemini IV space flight in 1965, one of the astronauts was found to have lost between one and twelve per cent of the bone mass in his hands and feet after only four days. The subsequent flight of Gemini V showed losses of more than twenty per cent. Recent research studies have shown the importance of exercise in combating osteoporosis.

The spine

The spine supports the head, ribs, shoulders and arms. It provides a safe pathway for the spinal cord, from which the motor and sensory nerves enter and exit at each vertebral level.

But if this were all it had to do, there would be no reason for its distinctive shape. By definition a straight line cannot bend. The spine is shaped so that we can bend, turn, walk, run, jump, skip, swing, swim.

But at birth we possess only two of the spine's four curves. Unlike Athene, we don't spring forth fully formed.

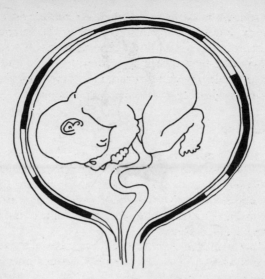

In the womb the baby lies curled like a cat, the primary curves already defined.

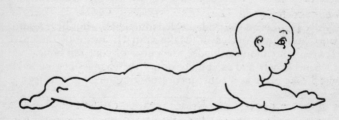

During its first six months of life, the child, lying in its cot, lifts its head to see through the bars. This is the first of the secondary curves – the cervical.

EXERCISE: Lie on your stomach, resting your nose on the floor, arms by your side. Raise your head and look around you. Repeat several times. Feel how the weight of the head brings about a change in the shape of the neck.

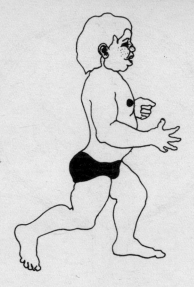

The second – the lumbar – develops when the child learns to stand upright and begins to walk.

EXERCISE: Lie on your side, curled into a ball, arms bent against your chest, head tucked in. Make yourself aware of the curve between your shoulder blades, the curve of your tail bone.

Uncurl slowly and as you do, notice the changes in your spine which take place as a consequence of straightening your legs.

Though the spine develops its distinctive shape initially out of a need to support the head and adjust to the upright stance, thereafter it is involved in all the movements of the arms and legs.

The spine is made up of twenty-four stacked joints – vertebrae – plus between eight and ten fused joints in the sacrum and coccyx.

Despite regional variations, vertebrae share the same basic pattern: a body to which an arch is tacked on to form a space

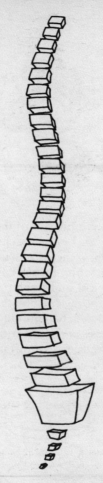

The spine

for the spinal cord. On either side of the arch are two projections called transverse processes and, at the back, a tail or spinous process. At the top and bottom of the arch there are also two articular processes for the articulation of each vertebra with the one above and the one below.

Typical vertebra

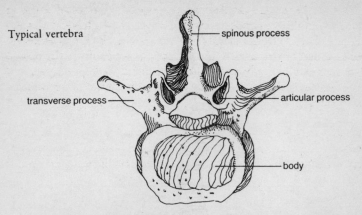

spinous process

transverse process

articular process

body

In between, making up a quarter of the spine's length, are the vertebral discs – little cushions attached to the body of the vertebra. Like the vertebra, they are shaped according to the job they have to do. For instance, they are thicker at the front than at the back in the cervical and lumbar regions to give greater flexibility, while in the thoracic region they are of even thickness throughout. But, subjected to continuous pressure, they lose some of their springiness and need a night's sleep to recover. When you get out of bed in the morning, you are fractionally taller than when you got into it.

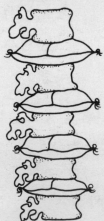

Discs imagined as cushions
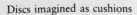

The vertebrae are divided into groups. Members of a group share a common purpose rather than identical physical characteristics. Each vertebra is shaped according to the kinds of movement to be carried out by the group. As we look at the design of the cervical, the thoracic and the lumbar vertebrae, you will see how their idiosyncrasies determine what kind of movement can be undertaken.

Cervical vertebrae Supporting the head are the seven small cervical vertebrae with their forked tails, which give a secure attachment to the ligament helping to nail the head to the trunk.

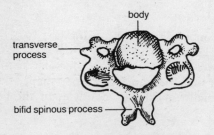

Cervical vertebra – upper surfaces

In addition, their transverse processes face inward and downward and so allow the neck great flexibility, especially at the back.

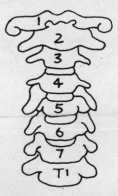

Cervical vertebrae as seen from behind

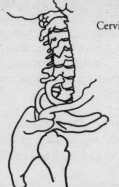

Cervical vertebrae – side view

EXERCISE: Look at the drawing, in particular at the angle of the transverse processes. Bend your head forward and back and sideways.

Of the seven, the most distinctive are the first two – the atlas and the axis. Unlike any other vertebra, the atlas has no body but is shaped like a ring to match the opening at the base of the skull. At either side, there are two kidney-shaped depressions into which the small knuckles or condyles of the head fit to make a joint.

EXERCISE: Imagine your head is supported by two little hands at the base of the skull. Nod gently. There is only the most rudimentary spinous process on the atlas so as not to interfere with the movement of the head.

Underneath, the axis (which more closely resembles other vertebrae) thrusts a finger through the ring of the atlas, thus forming another joint though of a different kind.

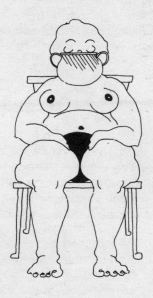

EXERCISE: Sit down. Imagine the lower half of your head as a bowl with handles where your ears are. The bowl is full of water. Without spilling a drop, turn your head first to the left and then to the right. This is the action of the head and atlas rotating around the finger of the axis.

Joints (the junction between two bones) run the gamut from the fixed to the freely movable and are further classified according to the shape of the bones concerned. The one between the atlas and the head is usually called a hinge joint, but a look at the shape of the surfaces to be joined suggests that the definition is unsatisfactory. However, that given to the joint of the atlas and axis – a pivot – is entirely satisfactory.

Thoracic vertebrae Larger than the cervical, the thoracic vertebrae support the ribs in protecting the lungs, heart, stomach, liver and spleen, and consequently have less need for flexibility. From the third downwards, their spinous processes partly overlap, which significantly limits the kind of back-bending that would have rendered the soft organs inside the rib cage vulnerable to attack, once upon a time.

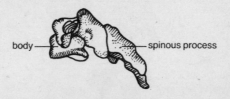

body —————   ————— spinous process

EXERCISE: Bend forward and back – feel how the spinous processes combine to stop you bending back.

Lumbar vertebrae The strongest and thickest vertebrae in the spine are the five lumbar vertebrae, for obvious reasons. Because of the variation in the depth of the discs, bending forward should be relatively effortless but the degree of back-bend is determined by the length of the spinous processes and the depth of the lumbar and sacral curves.

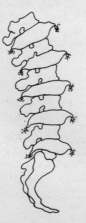

EXERCISE: Bend forward, imagining each vertebra resting on a little cushion. Bend back, bearing in mind the way the spinous processes stick straight out.

Sacrum Roughly triangular in shape, the sacrum is wedged between the two hip bones to bear the combined weight of the spine and head. Occasionally the fifth lumbar vertebra fuses with it. At its bottom edge, it joins up with the coccyx, formed by the fusion of between three and five tiny vertebrae.

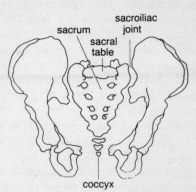

The sacrum articulates with the spine in the sacral table by means of a disc, to form the lumbosacral joint, and with the two hip bones, forming the sacroiliac joints.

EXERCISE: Resting on all fours, on hands and knees, curl your tail bone under as though your coccyx was being drawn toward your chin. Your sacrum will of course move too.

The joint between the sacrum and spine (the lumbosacral joint) and those between sacrum and hip bones (the sacroiliac joints) allow a minimal gliding movement, as shown in the following exercises.

EXERCISE: Lie flat on your back on the floor, arms folded over chest, knees bent. Your knees should be in a line with your hips, your heels in a line with your knees, and your toes in a line with your heels.

Imagine a clockface on the floor in between your hip bones, in place of your sacrum. Lightly press down on the 12, the 6, 3 and 9. Now move round clockwise and then anti-clockwise. The movement will be small.

EXERCISE: Sit sideways on the floor, resting on one hip, knees bent and tucked up beside you. Try not to let the lumbar portion of the spine slump. Change sides.

The ligaments   The responsibility for keeping the vertebrae in line with one another lies with the ligaments – fibrous bands running up and down the entire length of the spine, inside and outside and in between. At least fifteen support the head.

Ligaments protect their joints by limiting movement. Once stretched, they never go back to their original length. Consequently they can't do their job adequately. (A point which dancers in particular, or any person who goes in for intensive stretching exercises, should bear in mind.)

Thus far, we have looked at the spine according to its layout, but there are no strict boundaries between one part and another. Each area has evolved to merge smoothly with the next so that the spine can function as a whole. This sense of the whole is important in terms of strength, efficiency, grace, harmony and alignment – for the relationship of one vertebra to another can only be seen in the context of the whole spine. However separate the parts may look on the page or in the lecture room, their importance lies in their particular contribution to the whole.

The following exercises are designed to increase this sense of the whole spine.

EXERCISE: Lie on your back on the floor with your arms above your head, legs straight and slightly open in an inverted V.

Flex your feet so that the back of your heel is planted firmly on the floor. With both feet, press down as though on an accelerator. Press and flex, press and flex until your body is rocking back and forth along the floor. Try to feel the connection between the beginning and ending of your spine.

EXERCISE: Still on the floor, bend your knees and take your arms out to the side, palms to the floor. Check the alignment of knees with hips, feet and heels.

Gently rub your back on the floor as though you had an itch – all the way up and down the spine, the way a bear rubs its spine against a tree.

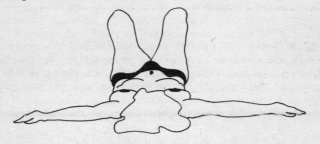

The pelvis

When we are born, the bones of the pelvis are not fused together but joined by cartilage. Complete ossification only takes place between the ages of fifteen and twenty-five.

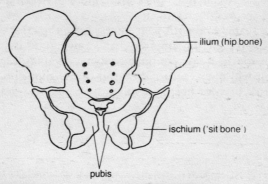

The six bones of the pelvis

The pelvis not only supports the spinal column, the head and arms, but also passes the weight on to the legs, and, via the long muscles which reach out from its bowl, connects the arms and legs to the centre of gravity which lies just in front of the sacrum (in the standing position), at roughly fifty-five per cent of the body's height.

EXERCISE: Sit in a chair with a hard, flat seat. Wriggle about until you can feel that you are sitting on bones rather than flesh. These are the flattened ends, about an inch long, of the pelvic bones – what the Americans refer to as the 'sit bones'. You will probably feel rather uncomfortable to begin with, especially if you are female and used to sitting with your legs crossed as mother told you to do. You will feel as though you are tipped a bit too far foward. However, your knees will not splay if you are seated correctly. On the contrary, they will feel as though they are falling towards one another. Because of the shape of the thigh bone, the knees are roughly in line with the 'sit bones'.

Transfer your weight from one 'sit bone' to the other, taking your head and spine with you as though you were cornering on a motor bike.

As with all other bony structures, connections (between sacrum and spine, between hip bones and spine, between pubis and ilium) are secured by ligaments.

Remain seated and with your fingers trace the crest of the hip bone – from the sacrum, up, round and down, until it disappears from your touch. If you continue probing, digging deep into the groin, you will come across the head of the thigh bone in the hip socket. Lift your heel and you will be able to sense it more easily.

EXERCISE: Sitting on the chair, on the 'sit bones', thighs pointed towards the mid-line, heels under the knees, toes in line with the heels, imagine the thighs and pelvis at right angles to one another, like the two leaves of a hinge with the pin connecting them running between the femoral (hip/thigh) joints.

Let your arms hang straight down. Imagine the hinge beginning to close – not much, only a little. Your body moves forward, your arms drop lower. Don't go any further than you can sustain the image.

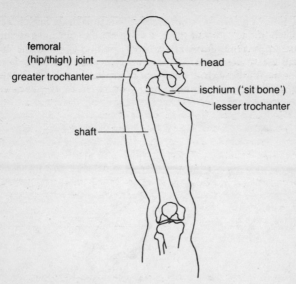

The femur or thigh bone as seen from the front. People often confuse the greater trochanter with the hip joint.

The joint between the thigh and the hip is described as a ball and socket joint, which allows a wider range of movement than that permitted by either the pivot or hinge. But in sitting, mobility is limited; only when standing or lying down are the restrictions on the joint's mobility lifted.

EXERCISE: Lie on your back on the floor, arms folded over your chest, knees bent, heels in line with knees, toes in line with heels. Draw your left knee towards a point midway between your nipples as if it were being drawn by a piece of elastic. Replace and repeat with the right.

EXERCISE: Same position as above. Lift the left knee up so that the foot clears the ground. Gently swing the lower leg from side to side like a pendulum. Replace and repeat on the other side. There should be little movement of the thigh. The lower leg acts like a lever to cause movement in the femoral joint.

EXERCISE: Same position once more. This time draw both knees towards your chest so that there is no strain on your back. Using your kneecaps as if they were brushes, paint a bow in the air. You will feel quite a lot of movement in your pelvis as your knees draw the bow, but don't try to stop it – go with it. As long as you keep your knees up over your chest, there will be no strain on your back.

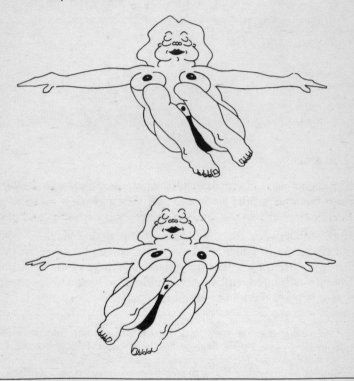

These three exercises will give you an idea of the range of movement afforded by the femoral joint.

The head of the thigh is kept in its socket by seven ligaments, of which the inverted Y ligament is the strongest. Characteristically it limits the backward extension of the leg, as well as securing the alignment of the pelvis on the legs. Damage to it, through over-stretching or doing sit-ups where the legs are in an extended position, endangers the very balance of the body.

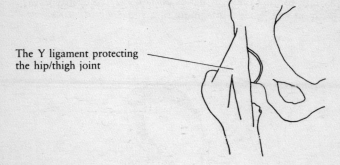

The Y ligament protecting the hip/thigh joint

The knee

The femur ends in two knuckles which rest on the table top of the tibia, one of the two bones of the lower leg, to form the knee joint – the largest and one of the most complicated joints in the body.

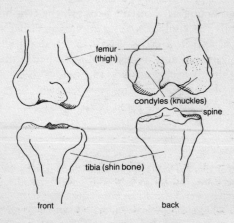

femur (thigh)

condyles (knuckles)

spine

tibia (shin bone)

front

back

Front and back view of the femur and tibia

From the front, the femur and tibia seem an unlikely couple; but looked at from behind, part of the reason for their successful partnership can be seen.

EXERCISE: Resting on your hands and knees, rock gently back and forth on your knees, imagining that you are on castors.

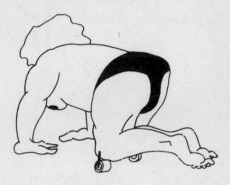

Further help is provided by cartilage which lines the bony surface of the tibia, acting as a buffer between the two bones. Stability is ensured by the vigilance of ligaments on either side as well as at the back, and in a cross-your-heart fashion within the joint itself. The kneecap acts as a shield, attached to the tendon of a group of thigh muscles above, and below to a ligament joined to the tibia. To prevent grating between joint, kneecap and floor, nature has provided fat pads both under and over the bone, giving us our own hassock.

EXERCISE: Lie on your stomach, bending both knees so that your lower legs are at right angles to your thighs. Make sure that your knees are roughly in line with your femoral sockets.

Alternately bend and straighten your legs on the ground. Don't lock your knees as you straighten, merely lay the shin on the ground.

The ankle

The ankle used to be classified as a hinge. It still is in many publications, but there are three bones involved in the ankle joint, which makes for something more complicated. The three bones are the talus (belonging to the foot) and the tibia and fibula (belonging to the leg), which enclose it on three sides.

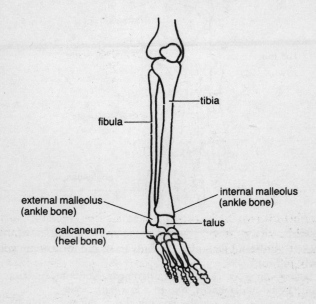

The ankle. What we call the ankle bones in reality belong to the tibia and fibula, the leg bones.

EXERCISE: Sit down on a chair and cross the right leg over the left. Flex the right foot. Imagine the talus as a golf ball. As you relax the foot, it rolls down a short incline before you catch it by flexing the foot once more.

EXERCISE: Same position, leg crossed, foot flexed. This time roll the golf ball round in a circular fashion.

The foot

Weight is transferred from the tibia to the talus and then via the heel bone to the rest of the foot.

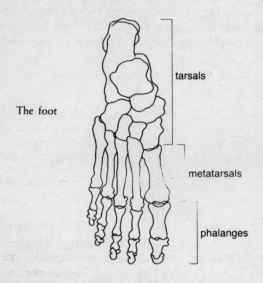

The foot

tarsals

metatarsals

phalanges

EXERCISE: Stand up and rock gently back and forward on your heels and toes.

Before you start, check your alignment. Knees under femoral joint, ankles under knees, toes in a line with heels.

Try and feel the weight flowing down through your body, collecting in the bowl of your pelvis, cradled on your legs; centred on knees and again on ankle joints, before connecting with the floor through your heel bones and spreading out to your toes.

There are twenty-six bones in the foot, arranged as a series of longitudinal and transverse arches.

EXERCISE: Sit on a chair, feet slightly apart. I like to think of the space between the instep and the ground as a kind of cave. Imagine someone painting the underside of one of your feet.

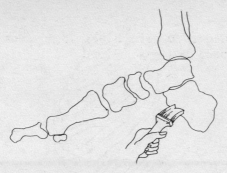

Starting at the inner edge of the heel, the brush is drawn up the highest arch of the instep and down to where the sole touches the ground. The second brush stroke begins at the centre of the heel and does not rise so high this time – the arch is lower. The final brush stroke commences at the outer edge of the heel and rises barely at all, virtually skimming the floor the entire length.

Because of the number of bones in the foot, the number of ligaments is correspondingly high – about fifty. Some are short, connecting neighbouring bones, while some, like the long plantar, reach from the underside of the heel to the toes (you will have felt it as you were rocking on your heels and toes), and others are used to support and restore the arch of the instep after each step. With its numerous ligaments, tendons and muscles, the foot is uniquely equipped for speed, flexibility and strength.

The rib cage

The rib cage is just that – a cage made up of twelve pairs of ribs curving protectively round the lungs and the heart, the stomach and the liver. At the back, they articulate with the thoracic vertebrae and in the front, the majority attach to the breast bone – a short, dagger-shaped bone.

The upper seven pairs attach to the breast bone and then three pairs join up with the seventh while the last two, the shortest, float free.

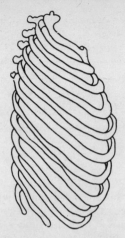

The rib cage – side view

A point worth bearing in mind is that all the ribs articulate with the thoracic vertebrae and the majority do it twice, for safety's sake. And at the front, the ribs are attached to the breast bone by a kind of pliable plastic called costal cartilage. All this means that though the rib cage can never be divorced from its support (the spine), it doesn't have to rely entirely on it but can, particularly with the aid of its muscular attachments, take the initiative.

EXERCISE: Lie on your back on the floor, knees bent; check alignment. Fold your arms over your chest so that your fingertips can touch the edge of the shoulder blades. Keeping your pelvis

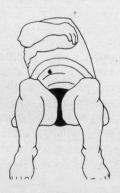

relatively still on the floor, roll the top half of your body from side to side, like a barrel. Roll your head in the same direction. There should be little noticeable movement of knees or pelvis.

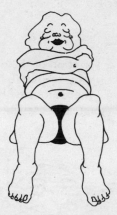

Continue rolling but, this time, keep your head still by staring fixedly at the ceiling.

Most people have only the vaguest idea of the shape of their ribs or where they begin and end. If you run your fingers down the back of your neck, you will come to a knob at the base which sticks out more than the rest – this is the vertebra prominens and is the last of the cervical vertebrae. The next one down is the first thoracic and articulates with the first of the ribs.

Leaving a finger pressed on the first thoracic, with your other hand find the top of your breast bone, where it joins up with the collar bones. Just underneath this meeting, the first ribs also join up with the breast bone.

Still with a finger on the first thoracic vertebra, and a thumb on the junction of breast bone and first rib, feel over the collar bone, in between the muscle cords, for the curve of that rib. Even though you probably won't be able to feel it unless you are very thin, you will get some idea not only of the narrowness of its circumference but also the way it slants downward from its attachment to the spine. As rib succeeds rib, the circumference not only widens (at least up to the seventh) and grows more elliptical but the angle between it and the vertebra becomes more acute. You can realise this by tracing with your fingers the outlines of the lower ribs.

The shoulder girdle

If you were asked for a description of the shoulder, what would you say? Round, small, singular or plural, bone or muscle? Part of the rib cage or arm, or synonymous with the shoulder blade?

Check your answers against the drawing.

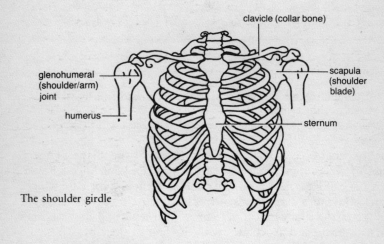

The shoulder girdle

The area generally referred to as the shoulder is the place where the collar bone, shoulder blade and arm meet. Strictly speaking, the shoulder girdle = 2 collar bones + 2 shoulder blades but, as you will have noticed, the arm is jointed to the shoulder blade and, consequently, any movement of the arm involves the shoulder blade and vice versa.

EXERCISE: Stand up and place one hand behind your back on the bottom-most tip of the opposite shoulder blade. Raise your free arm slowly in front of you, tracking the movement of the shoulder blade. Swing the arm behind you, then raise it above your head, still continuing to follow the movement of the shoulder blade.

EXERCISE: Same procedure but take the free arm out to the side.

Because the shoulder girdle is attached directly only at the front – to the breast bone – the shoulder blades in theory have unlimited freedom. But in reality they are kept firmly in their place by a multitude of overlapping muscles and by the positioning of the collar bones, whose handles act like a brace to push them back. 'Pull your shoulders back' should have been changed, a long time ago, to 'push your shoulders back'.

EXERCISE: Let the shoulders round, fall forward. Push them back with the handles of the collar bones.

EXERCISE: Lie on your back, knees bent. Raise both arms. With the left, reach towards the ceiling – the shoulder blade will be pulled away from the ground. Relax – the shoulder blade will drop back on to the floor. Repeat with the right arm.

EXERCISE: Same position on the floor, hands by your side.

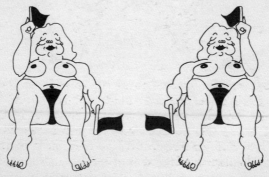

Imagine you have a flag in each hand. Raise the right arm so that it is above your head on the floor (don't force it if you can't touch the floor). As you start to bring it back, raise the left, and so on.

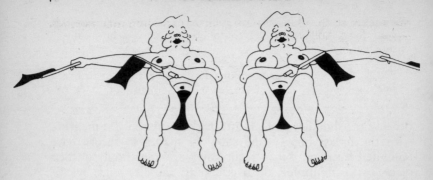

EXERCISE: Same position on the floor, arms out to the side. Fold one arm over your chest then return it to the floor. As you open, the other arm folds, etc.

EXERCISE: Same position, arms raised to the ceiling. To begin with, draw small circles in the air with the fingertips, then make them a little bigger and a little bigger until your arms are describing a large circle – touching the floor at the side, above your head, and crossing in front of your trunk. Reverse the circle and gradually decrease its size until you end up where you started.

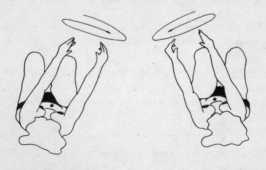

The arm/shoulder joint, like that of the hip and thigh, is of the ball and socket variety, but there the resemblance ends. The shoulder girdle, unlike the pelvis, has few responsibilities. It supports no weight other than that of the arms, consequently the head of the humerus (the upper arm) is hardly recessed in the socket at all. This allows the arms a freedom that would be irresponsible in the legs.

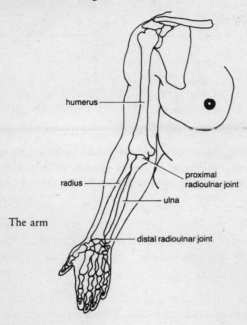

humerus

proximal
radioulnar joint

radius

ulna

The arm

distal radioulnar joint

The forearm

The ulna on the little finger side and the radius on the thumb side articulate with the upper arm at the elbow. The ulna and the radius articulate with each other below the elbow and at the wrist.

EXERCISE: Lie on your back, knees bent, arms out to the side, palms facing the ceiling. Bend and straighten your lower arms. This is the movement of the true hinge. When you bend your arms your palms should be facing one another.

EXERCISE: Stand up, arms by your side. Without moving your upper arm, turn your palms to face front. Place your other hand round your elbow so that you can feel radius and ulna articulating with each other.

EXERCISE: Bend the arm so that the palm faces the shoulder, then, turn it to face front. Place the other hand just above the wrist (about one and a half inches to two inches away) and you will feel the articulation.

Summary

● The alignment of the skeleton is a blend of nature and nurture. The more we understand of its nature, the better we shall be at nurturing.

● Bones are living structures, the cells within them continually at work, hindered or helped by what we eat, how we feel and what we do. The strength of our bones is, in part, a result of how much we use them.

● The spine is a series of joints, more capable of bending forward than back because of the shape of its spinous processes with only the neck designed to bend back easily. Gymnasts beware.

● The weight of the head and spine is supported by the pelvis, before being transferred to the legs. The bones of the pelvis do not ossify until the child has left school. Mothers in a hurry to send their young to ballet classes should ponder the implications.

● Ligaments exist to limit movement and if stretched cannot do their job properly, i.e. protect the joint.

● The ball and socket joints offer the greatest freedom of movement, and of these the arm and shoulder is the more emancipated. Unlike the hip/thigh, it has no responsibility other than itself.

● The arm is intimately connected to the shoulder blade – wherever the arm goes, the shoulder blade must follow.

● The shoulder blades are not meant to be pulled back but are braced in position by the collar bones.

● In the sitting position, the pelvis rests on the 'sit bones', the knees lined up with the deeply recessed hip/thigh joint.

● In the standing position, the pelvis rests on the joints, with the centre of gravity inside the bowl just in front of the sacrum – unless you have inordinately short legs coupled with an abnormally long torso.

● Weight is transferred through the knee to the ankle joint, where it is centred on the talus and thence to the heel and the toes.

● Gravity is an important factor in the alignment of the body. Allowing the weight of the head to rest on the atlas, letting the arms hang from the sockets of the shoulder blades instead of holding them up by the neck muscles, allowing the combined weight of head, spine and pelvis to rest on the hip/thigh joints, reduces tension and frees muscles for their creative work.

● If, for instance, the thigh is incorrectly lined up on the tibia, strain is placed on the ligaments of the knee – and the surrounding muscles may be called in to help. Like a 'good woman', a muscle will always step into the breach and help out. The problem is that unless the faulty alignment is corrected, what was temporary becomes permanent and the muscles will be forced into a situation where, by sustaining another, their own capabilities are severely diminished. It may go on unnoticed for years – apart from the occasional ache, twinge and spasm – but you don't need to be a student of tea leaves to know what the outcome will be.

CHAPTER 3
'Pick me up and lay me down'

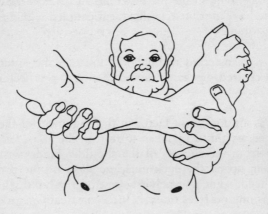

Skeletal muscles are often referred to as the 'engines of the body', producers of heat as well as locomotion. But the mechanical analogy bears little resemblance to the glistening lianas which shape our bodies in so many ways. Without them we could neither smile nor speak, pick our nose or plant a rose, copulate or procreate. Without them we would not be able to play the game, let alone stand up and fight. There would be no discussion as to whether it was better to be or not to be because we simply would not be able.

Attached to skin as well as bone, cartilage and ligament (either directly or indirectly), our skeletal muscles not only convey us, they convey our feelings and thoughts as well – our means of expression as surely as our means of transport.

Depending on whether you're British or American they make up either a quarter or a half of your body weight. Obviously, if they only account for a quarter of our weight, they cannot be said to materially shape our body. In other words, they are under-employed. Like people, muscles need to work. Without it, they atrophy.

Before we try and determine how much and what kind of work muscles need, we must get to know the work-force.

Skeletal muscle is made up of threadlike fibres which are elongated cells. Each is wrapped in connective tissue before being assembled into small bundles and wrapped again. The whole is then enclosed in a glistening sheath.

The fibres differ physiologically and biochemically but can be crudely divided into the quick and the slow. Like the tortoise and the hare, the slow members tire less easily than their dynamic partners. Fast-twitch fibres are commonly described as white and slow-twitch red, coloured by their extensive network of capillaries.

The fibres are grouped according to type and, together with their innervating motor nerve and motor neuron or cell, form what is called a motor unit. Not only does the number of fibres per unit vary (for instance the muscles that move the eye have less than ten fibres per unit, whereas those involved in a large limb may contain over one thousand) but also the number of motor units per muscle – the large muscles having many more than the small.

Though all the fibres in a unit contract simultaneously, to ensure smoothness in the action of the whole muscle, different motor units do not. It may look as if the whole muscle has contracted at once, but what the eye cannot see is that different motor units are discharging at different times.

Information is conveyed to the muscle fibres without a finger, so to speak, laid on them. The motor nerve carrying the charge stops short of the fibres, and the electrical transfer takes place across a minute gap through the release of a chemical substance either excitatory or inhibitory in nature.

Information from the muscle comes principally from spindle-shaped capsules lying between the fibres and from receptors in the tendons. Via the sensory nerves, the capsules inform the nervous system on changes in length and speed, and the receptors on force and tension.

There are thirty-one pairs of spinal nerves plus twelve cranial nerves. Though the sensory nerves enter by the back door of the spinal cord and the motor nerves leave by the front door,

Cross-section of spinal cord

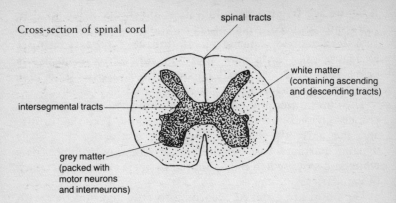

for the most part they travel the body together, only splitting up as they reach the muscle.

The grey horn-shaped core of the spinal cord is packed with motor neurons and the more numerous interneurons. The interconnections between the two form the basis of the integrative function of the spinal cord.

Immediately surrounding the core are fibres linking different spinal segments. These are the rails of the reflex response, involving a number of different spinal segments.

In the white matter enclosing the whole are more fibres running up and down, to and from centres in the brain. The majority of these cross in the area of the brain stem so that the right side of the body is principally controlled by units in the left hemisphere, and the left side by units in the right. However, a number of nerve fibres, both sensory and motor, do not make the crossing, preferring to keep solely to the right or left.

The interaction between the musculature and the nervous system forms an intricate communication network: between muscle and spinal cord, between spinal cord and muscle, between muscle and muscle, between muscle and brain, brain and muscle.

Admirable though the set-up is, its very complexity makes running the show anything but simple. This chapter is not a comprehensive tabling of every muscle in the body – only of a selected few. It is important to remember that muscles never work alone; it takes at least two, working in opposition, to operate a joint. Even the simplest movement attracts a crowd.

In the main, short muscles are concerned with fine movement, leaving posture to the long. This, however, is not the case with the neck muscles, which not only concern themselves with bending and tilting and turning the head but also with the balance of the head on the trunk.

Muscles of the neck

The fat semispinalis capitis and splenius capitis are both involved in straightening the head, but only the splenius capitis turns it.

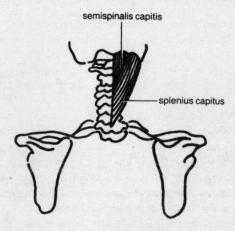

semispinalis capitis

splenius capitis

The action of bending forward is complicated by the weight of the head. As it tips forward, the muscles at the back of the neck put the brake on, rather like paying out a rope.

EXERCISE: Using that image, bend the head forward and to straighten, wind in the rope.

EXERCISE: Place your hands over the areas covered by the two splenius capitis. Turn the head from left to right so that you can feel the action of the muscles.

At the front of the neck, the sternocleidomastoids are like guy ropes securing the head to collar bones and breast bone. In movements such as bending forward, the two sternocleidomastoids act in unison, but in turning they act in opposition.

Sternocleidomastoids

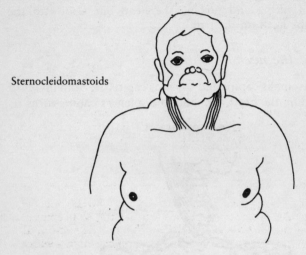

EXERCISE: Look in the mirror. You will notice a dimple just above the breast bone and between the two thongs of muscle. With your fingers, trace the thongs up to where they attach to the bones behind the ears. Turn your head from left to right and watch how the muscles work in opposition.

EXERCISE: Lie on your back and lift your head off the floor. Place one hand on the front of your neck to feel the muscles shorten as you lift.

Muscles of the shoulder girdle

Superimposed on the muscles at the back of the neck, like a starfish embroidered on the back, is the trapezius. Involved in movements of the shoulders as well as in raising the arms, its fibres are capable of working independently of each other as well as together. Experiment for yourself.

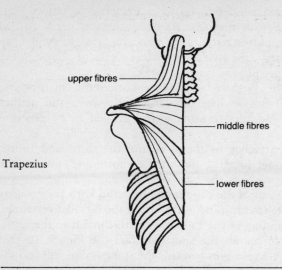

upper fibres

middle fibres

Trapezius

lower fibres

EXERCISE: Raise your shoulders — upper fibres. Pull the shoulder blades towards one another — lower and middle fibres. Lie on your stomach on the floor, legs together, arms by your side. Raise your head, neck and shoulders off the floor — whole muscle.

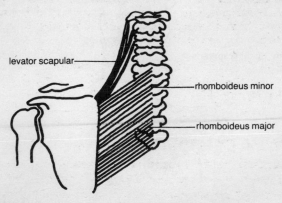

levator scapular

rhomboideus minor

rhomboideus major

Underneath the trapezius lie the muscles which connect the shoulder blades to the spine — the levators and the rhomboids.

If any muscles could be said to characterise a nation, then these are the British muscles. At some time in every British child's life, 'shoulders back' and 'stand up straight' will have rung in their ears – the two most useless pieces of advice in the English language, physiologically speaking.

Positioning the shoulder blades is the work of the collar bones; muscles should not be used for structural work, and neither the rhomboids nor the levators were intended to be postural muscles.

The levator attaches to the atlas and the third and fourth cervical vertebrae. Imagine the muscle shortening, pulling the shoulder blade towards the back of the head.

Look at the slant of the rhomboid fibres and with your fingers feel for the vertebra prominens, the last of the cervical vertebrae. This is the beginning of the rhomboid's attachment to the spine. Keeping your finger on the spot, contract the muscle so that your shoulder blade moves towards the spine – you will feel the muscle tense.

The underside of the shoulder blade is cushioned by the subscapularis. It is attached, like the trapezius, to the upper arm, which allows the little boy in the playground or the *agent de police* to twist your arm behind your back without breaking it off.

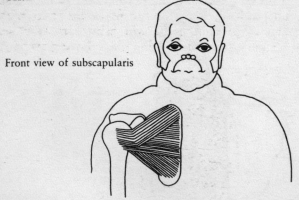

Front view of subscapularis

It is one of four muscles forming a protective cuff around the shoulder/arm joint; the others in the group are the supraspinatus, the infraspinatus and teres minor. These are the muscles which prevent the heavy shopping bag or suitcase from pulling your arm out of its socket.

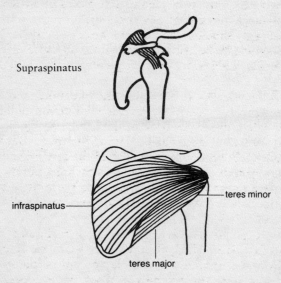

Supraspinatus

infraspinatus

teres minor

teres major

Like a short sleeve, the deltoid curves round the shoulder. Its fibres work independently (the posterior fibres are active with the infraspinatus in preventing the arm being torn from its socket) or as a team — best illustrated in the following exercise.

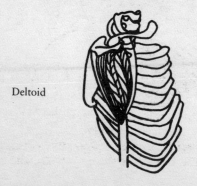

Deltoid

EXERCISE: Bend the arm so that the fingers rest on top of the shoulder. Swing the arm in a backward arc. Reverse and swing in a forward arc.

In walking, the posterior fibres are largely responsible for the backward swing of the arm, while the latissimus dorsi is involved in the forward position.

Though not a member of this group of muscles, the latissimus dorsi provides a link between upper and lower extremities, between shoulder and pelvic girdles. Place the drawing in front of you and raise your arms high above your head. Follow the muscle as it rises obliquely up from the sacrum to its attachments on the arms.

Latissimus dorsi

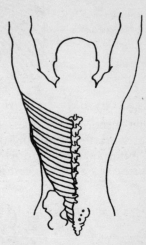

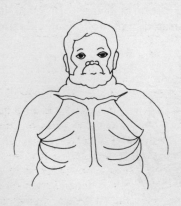

Spread across the chest are the body builder's friends – the pectorals – also very popular with cricketers and golfers.

Pectoralis major

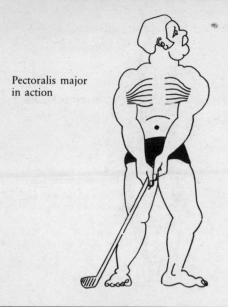

Pectoralis major
in action

EXERCISE: Place the right hand on the left half of the chest –
heel of the hand on the breast bone, thumb touching the collar
bone and, if your fingers are long enough, finger tips on the arm.
Raise the left arm out to the side and swing it in front of you
and across, just as if you were batting or playing a golf stroke.
Repeat on the other side.

Muscles of the spine

The complexity of the spinal column makes for an equally
complex arrangement of muscle. This, in turn, makes it difficult
to state categorically which does what. Generally speaking, the
short deep muscles are concerned with stability between vertebra
and vertebra, while the long deep muscles are concerned with
the stability of the spine as a whole. Sitting or standing in a
relaxed position makes few demands of either, depending on the
alignment of the trunk, of course. Bending, whether forwards,
backwards or sideways, immediately engages them.

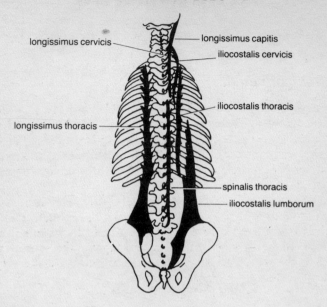

longissimus cervicis —   — longissimus capitis

                   — iliocostalis cervicis

                   — iliocostalis thoracis

longissimus thoracis —

                   — spinalis thoracis

                   — iliocostalis lumborum

The deep muscles of the back – the erector spinae – are divided into three columns: the iliocostalis, the longissimus and the spinalis, each with a lower, middle and upper part. Those of the iliocostalis are known as the lumborum, thoracis and cervicis, while those of the other two are known as the thoracis, cervicis and capitis.

EXERCISE: Lie on your stomach, arms by your side, legs together. Lift your head, arms and legs.

In bending forward, gravity exerts its pull and the spinal muscles behave like the neck muscles when faced with a similar situation. This time, though, the odds are too great and once the trunk passes the half-way mark, they hand over the job to the ligaments. When fully bent over, we are literally hanging from our ligaments.

Despite the combined strength of all the spinal ligaments, it's not the sort of position in which to lift a box of groceries or move about making the bed. In the circumstances, the only safe movement is *up*. Not even the abdominal muscles are active.

Abdominal muscles

Nowhere in the body is evolution more clearly to be seen than in the abdomen. Whereas, in the animal, the belly faced the ground, relatively well protected from sudden attack, in the upright stance it was exposed and vulnerable. To compensate, the abdominal muscles evolved their own protective clothing – a kind of corset.

First, a thin layer is wrapped round the belly, tendons meeting centre front to form a seam. The next layer, like so many tacking stitches, runs on either side of it from the ribs to the pubis. The tendons of the first layer form a backing for the second and those of the third and fourth form a covering to make a firm front panel – a synthetic girdle.

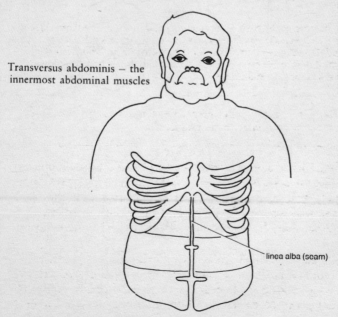

Transversus abdominis – the innermost abdominal muscles

linea alba (seam)

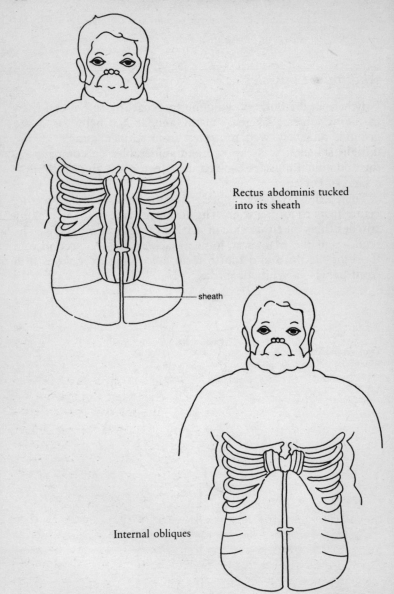

Rectus abdominis tucked
into its sheath

sheath

Internal obliques

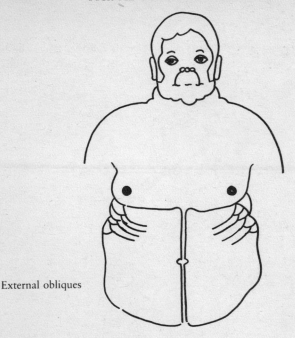

External obliques

Like the spinal muscles, the abdominals show little activity when we are sitting or standing. The simplest though not the most aesthetic method of activating the internal and external obliques (the third and fourth layers) is to sit down and strain, making sure that the pelvis isn't tilted. Activation of the rectus abdominis (tacking stitches) has no such lavatorial connotation, you merely cough. Place a hand over an area of the muscle and try it.

Because of the strain on the lumbar spine and on the Y ligaments of the hip/thigh sockets, sit-ups should only be done with the legs bent. After the first 45 degrees the abdominals are only mildly active. So, if you are addicted to sit-ups, come up off the ground only so far as your head, arms and shoulders clear the floor. To activate the obliques, come up aiming the right arm towards the left knee.

The diaphragm

In humans, the main respiratory muscle is the diaphragm. Which other muscles are involved and the extent of their involvement

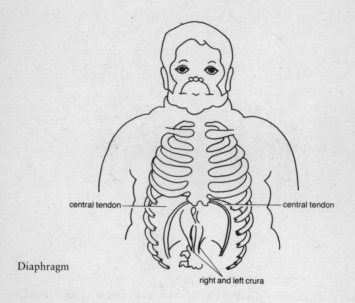

central tendon —————   ————— central tendon

Diaphragm

right and left crura

is less certain, though the use of electromyography to measure activity in muscles during respiration has thrown light on many a murky corner.

What we do know absolutely is that the diaphragm is made up of muscle fibres radiating from a central tendon, attached by muscular slips to the breast bone, lower six ribs and the upper lumbar vertebrae, but functioning as a whole. Altogether it forms an umbrella over the liver and stomach and other organs, higher on the right than on the left because of the liver's greater size.

EXERCISE: With your fingers trace the origins of the muscle. Start at the tip of the breast bone. Breathe in and out.

Now dig your fingers under the relevant ribs – the seventh to tenth. Breathe in and out. Now find the tips of the eleventh and twelfth ribs. Breathe in and out.

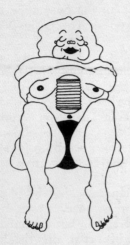 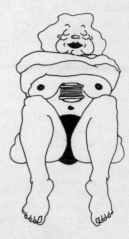

Imagine the diaphragm as an accordion. As you breathe in, it expands; as you exhale, it contracts.

What you will not have felt is the flattening of the central tendon which takes place as you breathe in. This downward action draws air in through the nose and into the lungs where the exchange of oxygen and carbon dioxide takes place.

During quiet breathing, the central tendon drops unspectacularly – about 1.5 cm – but in deep breathing it plummets between seven and ten cms.

EXERCISE: Take a normal breath and imagine a lift descending just one floor and coming back up again. Next, take a deep breath and imagine the lift descending to the basement.

Like rubbish, myths have accumulated around the working of the diaphragm. None causes more confusion than the theory that it is mobilised by the abdominal muscles – in particular the rectus abdominis.

By placing a hand under the breast bone, you are advised to breathe in by pushing against your hand. Then, keeping the ribs extended, you are told to push the air out by pulling in the rectus abdominis (the one you've just pushed out). This is called 'breathing with your diaphragm'.

However, there is no evidence that, in healthy people, the abdominal muscles are involved in inspiration, other than in a reflective capacity; and little to suggest that they are under the control of the respiratory centre in the brain stem. What is more, recent evidence shows that the diaphragm, far from needing the services of the rectus abdominis or any other of the abdominals to activate it, mobilises a full quarter of a second before inspiration occurs and before any of the accessory muscles are involved.

It is easy to see how the confusion arose, just by placing a hand in the space underneath the breast bone. Every time you take a breath, there is movement to be felt. But the movement is caused by the displacement of the liver et al, after the descent of the central tendon and the flattening out of the diaphragm; just as the diaphragm is itself affected by the state or position of the stomach and liver after a heavy meal or when lying or sitting down.

Only in forceful breathing out are the abdominal muscles employed. Normally breathing out is considered passive; what slight activity has been recorded is described as a kind of braking action in response to the elastic recoil of the lungs. If the abdominals are used, however, the breath can be expelled quickly.

EXERCISE: Breathing in, generally, takes less time than breathing out. For practice, breathe in for two counts and out for three.

This time, breathe in for two but expel the air in one.

In normal exhalation, added braking power is given to the diaphragm by the quadratus lumborum, a muscle more normally seen in action in the rocking movements of children. Test for yourself. Sit on a hard chair and rock from 'sit bone' to 'sit bone'.

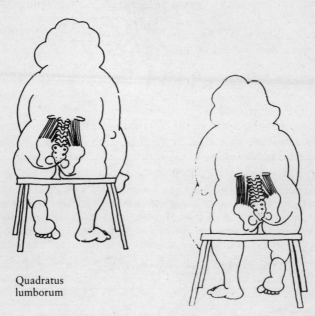

Quadratus
lumborum

Muscles of the pelvis and legs

One of the longest muscles in the body – the iliopsoas – is also one of its principal postural muscles. As plain psoas, the muscle leaves the lumbar spine to slide inside the hip bone where it picks up the iliacus muscle. They continue, under the name of iliopsoas, to attach on the inside of the thigh.

As befits a prime postural muscle, it is active in stabilising the hip/thigh joint but, on account of its depth, is inaccessible except to the imagination.

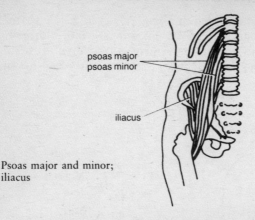

Psoas major and minor;
iliacus

You can sense its action in the following exercise.

EXERCISE: Lie on your back on the floor, arms folded loosely
over your chest, knees bent at approximately a 90-degree angle.
Check the alignment of knees with hip/thigh sockets and of big
toes and inside edge of heels. Breathe in, and on the exhalation
bring your knee towards the mid-line of your chest; your toes
are the last to leave the floor and the first to return as you replace
your leg. Repeat on the other side. If you place a hand on the
lumbar spine you will feel the muscle working.

The iliacus can best be sensed during the later phase of sit-ups
(the last 45 degrees). Try it but make sure you do it with knees
bent.

The next group of muscles all have one thing in common:
they are our wheels, whether they take us dancing or to the
office.

The buttocks are principally moulded by the three gluteals –
gluteus maximus (about an inch thick), medius and minimus.
Though they are not considered postural muscles, it is generally
accepted that they help to keep the pelvis stable during walking,
preventing it from sagging on the transfer of weight.

Place both hands on the buttocks and walk around the room
until you are familiar with the action of the muscles.

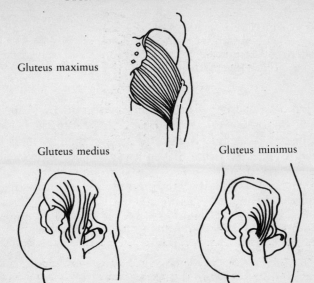

Gluteus maximus

Gluteus medius

Gluteus minimus

They also combine with the hamstrings (three in number) to lift your leg behind you.

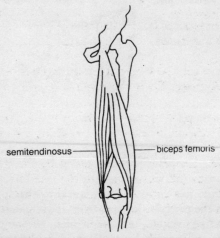

semitendinosus——— ———biceps femoris

Two of the three hamstrings: semitendinosus and biceps femoris. Semimembranosus, the other hamstring, lies in front of semitendinosus.

EXERCISE: Place your hands on your buttocks again and lift
first the left and then the right leg. Change the position of the
hands to cover the area of the three hamstrings and repeat, lifting
the leg off the ground behind you.

Lifting the leg in front is principally the job of the quadriceps
femoris – as its name suggests, a four-headed muscle. It is very
powerful and thought to possess three times more strength than
the hamstrings. Over-enthusiastic use produces a thigh like a
stocking packed with rocks. You can experiment yourself.
Straighten a leg and lift it off the ground in front of you, placing
a hand on the muscle. Tense very hard and then reduce the
tension to the level needed to hold up the leg and no more.

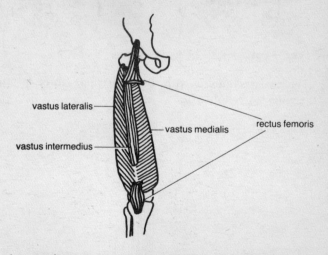

vastus lateralis

vastus medialis

rectus femoris

vastus intermedius

Quadriceps femoris (showing rectus femoris cut back to reveal the three
vasti)

It would make for clarity if one could say that the muscle on
the outside of the thigh – the tensor fascia lata – lifted it to the
side and that the muscles on the inside, the adductor group
(longus, brevis and magna) returned it. Unfortunately, while the
tensor fascia lata undoubtedly does lift the leg to the side (try

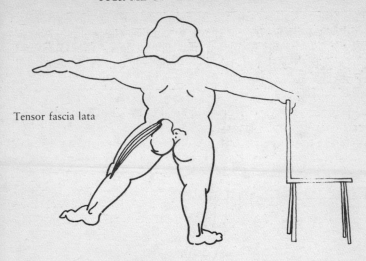

Tensor fascia lata

it), the role of the adductors in returning it is questionable, unless against resistance. They are, however, active whenever you bend your knee as you will feel if you grab the inside of your thigh.

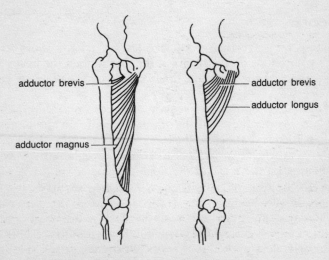

adductor brevis

adductor magnus

adductor brevis

adductor longus

The title of longest muscle in the body goes to the sartorius, the tailor's muscle. If you place a hand at the point where it crosses over to the inside of the thigh above the knee and straighten the leg out in front of you, you will be able to feel part of the muscle at work.

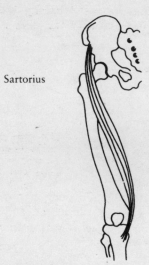

Sartorius

Before we leave this group of muscles, take a short stroll. Place your hands on the fronts of the thighs, then the backs and sides, and feel the constant flow of activity. Walking is great exercise.

With one exception, the activity of the calf and shin muscles is related to the foot – all but three originate on the bones of the lower leg and attach to the foot. Two of the three exceptions – the gastrocnemius and its accessory, the plantaris – while originating on the back of the thigh terminate, via the Achilles tendon, on the heel so that they too are involved in what happens to the foot.

Underneath them, the soleus works hard to stabilise the leg on the foot and, because of the large number of sensory receptors in the muscle, is remarkably well-informed.

It is important to realise that what happens in the foot is a direct result of what has happened elsewhere in the body. Wearing high heels, for instance, changes the centre of gravity and increases activity amongst the calf muscles with subsequent changes in the foot. Even as little as a five-degree swing backwards or forwards produces increased activity in the muscles of the calf and shin. Experiment yourself. Stand up and move your

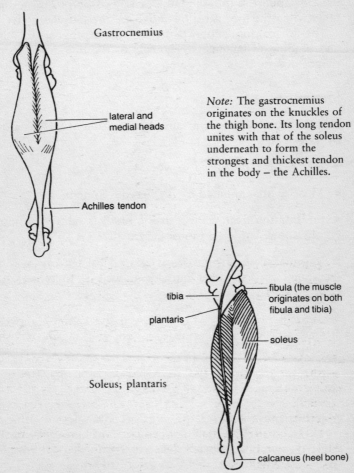

Gastrocnemius

lateral and medial heads

Achilles tendon

Note: The gastrocnemius originates on the knuckles of the thigh bone. Its long tendon unites with that of the soleus underneath to form the strongest and thickest tendon in the body – the Achilles.

tibia

plantaris

fibula (the muscle originates on both fibula and tibia)

soleus

Soleus; plantaris

calcaneus (heel bone)

head – to the side, look over your shoulder, up at the ceiling – keeping your attention centred on the soles of your feet as they reflect the changes happening some distance away. Now bend over, just a little, to the side, to the front, to the back. This time the changes are a bit more noticeable.

Support of the arches of the foot has traditionally been accorded to the muscles, but electromyography has shown muscle support in the standing-at-ease position to be negligible. Only when the foot is on the move are the muscles active.

The normal foot supports itself by the arrangement of bones and binding of ligaments. The role of the muscles is to move that structure.

Summary

Skeletal muscles are our means of expression as well as a means of transport.

- Like people, they need to work.

- Muscles are animated by the nervous system.

- Information from centres in the brain is relayed to muscles via the spinal cord and motor nerves.

- Information from muscles is relayed by sensory nerves via the spinal cord to other muscles as well as to centres in the brain.

- Muscles are never solitary – even the simplest movement attracts a crowd. It takes at least two, working in opposition, to control a joint.

- Generally speaking, short muscles concern themselves with fine movement, leaving postural work to the long.

- In the spine, however, the short deep muscles are principally concerned with the stability between vertebra and vertebra, while the long muscles are concerned with the stability of the spine as a whole.

- *Touching your toes can be dangerous*. When fully bent over, the spinal muscles clock out and you are left hanging from your ligaments.

- The diaphragm is the major respiratory muscle in the body. There is no evidence that the abdominal muscles are involved in inspiration, though they may be utilised to exhale quickly.

- The abdominal muscles are a four-layer corset. Activating them is easiest done by straining and coughing. Because of the strain on the lumbar spine and on the Y ligaments of the hip/ thigh sockets, sit-ups should always be done with the knees bent. *Only in the first 45 degrees of sit-ups are the abdominals fully active.*

- In the standing position, the arches of the foot are maintained by the bones and ligaments.

- When the body is well balanced, standing, sitting or lying evokes little muscular activity. Tiredness does not come from sitting or standing for long periods but from a badly balanced body. Even the so-called postural muscles are not made to do structural work.

- *No matter where they are, muscles are not there to prop you up but move you on.*

CHAPTER 4
'Is it for all time or simply a lark?'

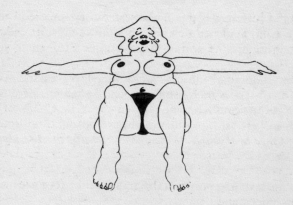

Human skills, in contrast to animal skills, take longer to develop because the co-ordination and integration they require are made more difficult by the complexity of the human nervous system. Though we think of ourselves as undoubtedly superior, that superiority is based on the fact that we can talk, think, write and paint. It does not occur to us that we might also be superior in what are called 'motor', skills. And because it hasn't occurred to us, it comes as a surprise when some talented individual appears — an exception rather than the rule.

If we pause to consider the range and variety of our physical activity and the skills that are required, then our potential stares us in the face. Recognition of that potential is what this final chapter is about.

The human being acquires his basic skills, stage by ordered stage, during childhood. Growth occurs in spurts; the timing may vary but the order not. In between these spurts, the child develops expertise by trial and error. Unfortunately, children are neither equal nor are they masters of their own destinies, and many of the stages are insufficiently grounded before the next has arrived. Poor co-ordination between hand and eye, between right and left sides of the body, between upper and lower extremities accompany the child into adulthood. By the time he or she comes of age, debt is more normal a state than credit.

Yet the human being is nothing if not adaptable. The disadvantages of childhood can be turned round, faults righted, the deficit made up. We can go back over the stages and get them right. We can make sense of the past and put it to better use.

There are many systems of exercise which, like Czerny, become a way of life; not the means to an end but the goal itself. The exercises which follow are not of that order. By working through our own developmental pattern we can see for ourselves, at first hand, the stages we muddled through, skipped over. Using the mirror of self-awareness, we can re-pattern our movement. The exercises are not for life, but to be picked up and put down when needed. Repetition for repetition's sake is for the robot not the human body, a technique for getting things right – 'if at once you don't succeed' and all that. But once you have, its value plummets. The human body, unlike a machine, is incapable of exact repetition. Continued practice is as likely to set the body going in the wrong direction as to keep it up to the mark.

Some of the exercises are one-offs, but most are members of a group, variations on a simple move. To begin with, limit yourself to one particular group. Only when you have mastered all the exercises in the group and can perform the moves fluently is it time to take on board the next. After that, it is up to you to use them when you find it necessary. You may well develop variations of your own. Exercises carry no copyright, belong to no one teacher – we all learn from one another, adding to what we already know, adapting, changing. I would like to think that these exercises are a beginning rather than an end.

To concentrate the mind, forget that you have a speech to write, an estimate to prepare, that your daughter hasn't a clean school blouse, or that your mother-in-law is about to arrive, and lie on the floor on your back with your knees bent, feet flat. (Always check on the alignment of hip/thigh joints, knees, heels, big toes before you start.) Fold your arms loosely over your chest so that your elbows are resting on top of one another in the middle of your chest (this rather depends on the length of your arms and/or the amplitude of your breasts). Close your eyes and breathe in and out deeply ten times without losing track of the count. If you do, go back to the beginning.

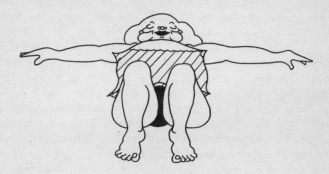

Now open your arms out to the side and imagine your trunk is a pillow full of water, the four corners of which are the two shoulder/arm joints and the two hip/thigh joints. Breathe in before rolling the pillow (keeping the corners in alignment with each other) on to its side. Consider the water level – your breath should have given out as you come on to your side. Breathe in again and begin the roll back, noting how the water spreads itself over the width and length of the pillow.

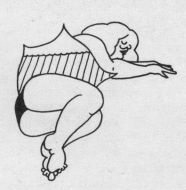

At first you won't know what to do with your arms. Don't try to do anything with them, let them find their own way to the floor, to your trunk. Your shoulders and hips will also feel uncomfortable as you roll over. The more you allow yourself to feel the weight of the water slopping around inside your trunk, the more relaxed you will become.

These two exercises should precede any others.

Exercise 1

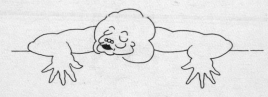

Lie on your tummy with your head turned to the right so that your left cheek is on the floor, arms as in the drawing. Breathe in as you lift your head; your shoulders should come off the floor as well, but not much. Look round you as you slowly turn your head from right to left. Breathe out as you lower your right cheek to the floor. Repeat the movement, noting the change in pressure in the cervical spine, in the area between the shoulder blades, in the lumbar spine.

Variation 1   Repeat the exercise, with the same breathing pattern, but this time your head, shoulders and upper chest are higher off the ground.

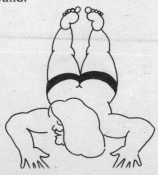

Variation 2   Go back to the original starting position, with your left cheek on the floor, but bring your elbows closer to your body so that weight can be taken on them. Lift your head and shoulders a little further off the ground and, turning to the right, peer towards your right foot as you breathe in. Your weight will be distributed between the left side of your body and your right elbow. Breathe out as you turn to repeat on the other side.

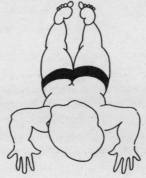

Variation 3   Exactly the same routine but with your head, chest and shoulders even further off the floor. As you turn to the right your right forearm will remain flat on the floor but your left arm will bend so that only your left hand is on the floor. The distribution of weight will be between the left side of your body and your right elbow as before, but you will have rolled further over on to the left side. Repeat on the other side.

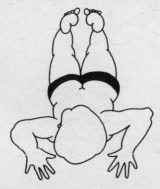

Exercise 2

Lie flat on your stomach once more, with head turned so that your right cheek is on the floor, arms as in the first drawing. Breathe in and bend your left leg so that the calf is at a 90-degree angle to the thigh on the floor. As you breathe out, replace it on the floor and bend the right. Notice the way the weight transfers to the right of the pelvis as you lift your left calf, and to the left as you lift your right calf. Change to left cheek and repeat.

Variation 1 Original starting position, breathe in once more as you bend left leg. On the breath out, lift your left thigh off the ground and roll over on to your right hip (keeping the upper part of the body on the floor) so that your left foot almost touches the ground on the far side of your right leg. Come back to the starting position and repeat several times until the movement is fluent, noticing the changes that take place in the spine. Repeat on the other side – make sure you turn your head so that your left cheek is on the floor when you use your right leg.

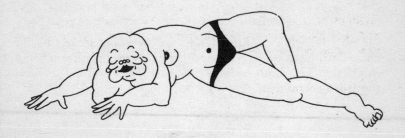

Variation 2 Same starting position – bend left leg, breathing in as you do. Repeat the preceding exercise – except that when your left foot touches down, push on the floor with your hands and come up to sitting, right leg straight out in front of you, left leg bent.

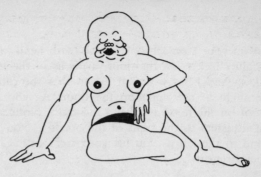

Repeat by going back the way you've come, taking the weight on your hands, rolling over your right hip and on to your abdomen. The aim of the exercise is to make it one smooth operation from beginning to end.

Exercise 3

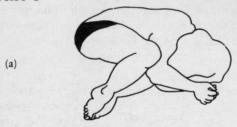

(a)

Lie on your left side, knees and arms bent and close to your chest. Breathe in before you start the exercise, and as you begin to exhale, curve both ends of the spine (head and tail) inward towards one another, as if your back was a bow. (a)

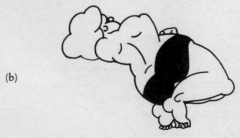

(b)

The movement is small — large only in the imagination. As you take another breath, arch your back, feeling the tail bone push down and back while your head describes a backward arc on the floor to pull your body flat before rolling over to your other side. Curl up on the exhalation and begin again. (b)

Variation 1 Lying on your back, arms relaxed and slightly above your head, bend your knees but not too close to your body.

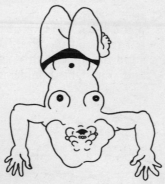

Breathe in and, on the out breath, let the weight of your thighs, particularly the left, pull the lower half of your body on to your left buttock so that your left leg is on the ground, but not your right. Feel the pull between the top of the spine and the tail bone. Breathe in, check that your left buttock is not tense, breathe out and bring your right leg, followed by your left, back up to the starting position. Repeat other side.

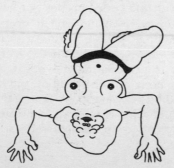

Variation 2   Lie on your back again, knees bent (not too close to your body), arms relaxed and slightly above your head. Breathe in and press down with your left foot on the floor so that your left buttock leaves the floor and your weight is tipped on to your right. The momentum takes you on to your front and from there, on to your back. Bend your knees, breathe in and press down with your right foot and repeat.

Variation 3   Lie on your back, arms horizontal to your body, knees bent up over your chest.

The intention is to roll the lower half of the body on to the left hip so that the left leg is on the floor, the right resting on top of it, leaving behind the upper half – shoulders, head and arms – flat on the floor (the right shoulder will not be entirely flat).

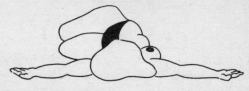

There will be those of you for whom this presents problems but do not force, only go as far as it is easy.

Don't do the exercise too slowly, keep it moving from side to side. The level at which the knees start off (say over the waist-line) must be maintained, particularly when the lower half is rolled over to the side.

Variation 4   Start in the curled-up position on your left side. As if you were going to yawn and stretch, open your right arm and place it on the floor, palm uppermost, so that your upper back is flat on the floor while your lower half remains on its side. As your right arm touches down, your right knee pulls the lower half of your body flat on the floor and over on to your right side, followed by your left knee. Your left arm follows on as soon as your left knee touches down and closes on your right. You are now lying curled up on your right side and ready to repeat the exercise.

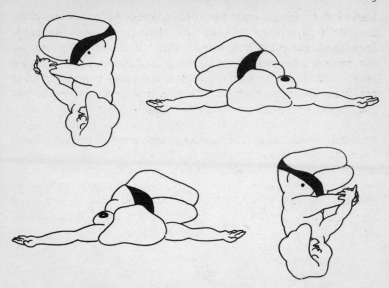

Variation 5 Start curled up on the left side. Breathe in as you arch back, but this time extend both arms and legs. Keeping your arms above your head, roll over on to your back and over on to your right side. Curl up and repeat.

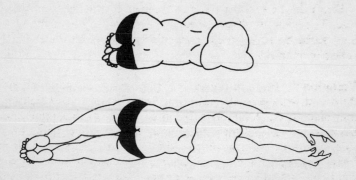

Variation 6 Lying on your back, arms relaxed and above your head, legs apart, cross your left leg over your right. As it crosses (the big toe aiming for the floor about eighteen inches to two

feet away from the little toe of the right foot) it will pull you
over on to your right side and then on to your front. Now, lift
the right leg and cross it over the left. The momentum set up
by the leg, as it crosses on its way to the floor, will roll you
over, first on to your side and then on to your back. Repeat
and then reverse, starting with the right leg crossing over the left.
Keep your legs straight and don't make a big deal of crossing the
leg. Don't, for instance, lift it high in the air – instead keep it
low, barely skimming the other leg. And don't anticipate the roll
by initiating it with the trunk, but let the leg be the instigator.

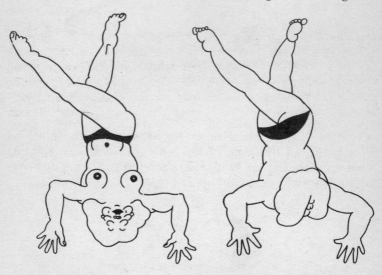

Variation 7   Begin the exercise as before – crossing left leg over
right and rolling on to your front – but then, instead of your
right leg, lift your right arm and at the same time roll onto your
left side and over on to your back. You will find it easier if you
keep some distance between your arms when they are on the
floor. Repeat before reversing.

By the time you have arrived at these last two variations, you
should have established a rapport with the floor so that you
now glide over rather than bump.

Variation 8 Lie on your back, knees bent, arms out to the side relaxed. Breathe in, and on the exhalation lift your head just a fraction off the floor and place it down a little way to the left. Breathe in, and on the exhalation bring it back to the centre. Repeat to the right.

Variation 9 Same as above except, this time, lift not only your head but also your shoulders off the floor. As you move to the left, your arms will be displaced. In both exercises, keep your eyes fixed on the ceiling so that it is the back of your head which is on the floor.

Variation 10 Same position except for the arms, which are placed straight out to the side. Breathe in and on the exhalation lift the head, shoulders and arms and place them down left of centre. The pelvis neither moves nor tilts though the torso is curved in the direction of the left. Breathe in and on the exhalation lift and bring the head and trunk back to centre. Repeat to the right.

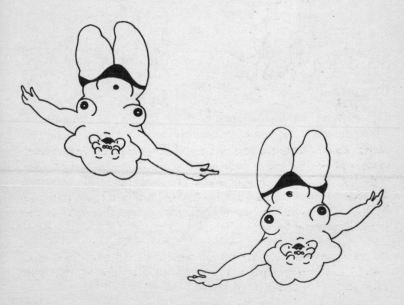

Variation 11   Same position as for Variation 8. Flex the left foot so that the toes come off the floor. Swivel on the heel and place the toes on the ground so that the whole foot is turned out. Flex the right foot, swivel, and place the toes down so that the foot is turned in. Raise the left heel off the ground and swivel, placing it down so that the left foot is turned in. Raise right heel, swivel, and place down so that the right foot is turned out. Continue until you can go no further. All the while, the pelvis remains on the ground but the action of the feet angle the pelvis to the left so that the left hip is closer to the spine than the right. Repeat the procedure to bring yourself straight and repeat to the right.

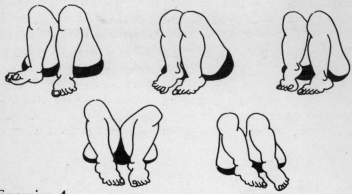

Exercise 4

This exercise and its variations should, ideally, be done on an uncarpeted floor. If you have no alternative but to work on the carpet, expect to move very little and don't repeat the exercises excessively.

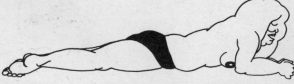

Lie on your front, legs straight, arms bent as in the drawing, hands in a fist. Breathe in, and as you exhale, press down on the floor with forearms and fists, lift head and chest a little way clear of the floor, and push yourself back. You will feel the abdominal muscles at work.

Stay where you are, don't adjust your arms. Breathe in and tuck your toes forward (as in the drawing). As you exhale, push your body forward from the toes. You should arrive back at the starting position. Repeat, making sure that you have got the breathing right, exhaling on the move, inhaling while stationary.

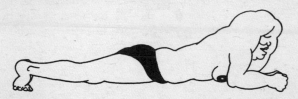

Variation 1 Lie on your stomach, legs straight. Bring the hands level with and close to the shoulders, spreading fingers out on the floor, palms flat. Breathe in and lift head, turning it to the right. Breathe out and bear down on the right hand and push the right side back. Adjust the position of the hands, turn the head to the left and push back with the left hand and forearm.

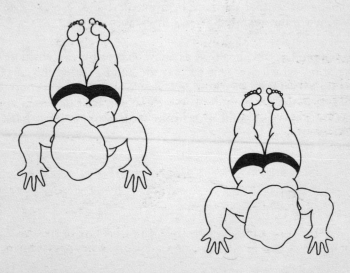

Variation 2   On your front, legs straight, hands close and level with the shoulders. Tuck your toes forward and push your body forward with first the left and then the right toes.

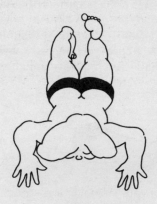

Variation 3   This exercise is only possible on an uncarpeted floor. Lying on your front, lay both hands, palms down, a little way in front of you. Breathe in and on the exhalation bear down and pull yourself forward. Repeat, each time adjusting your hands so that they are in front of you. If the exercise is easy, reach out with the arms a little more.

Variation 4   Same position as above except for the position of the arms, which are bent so that the hands, curled into a fist, are on a level with the shoulders. Inhale and rest the feet on the toes, as in the drawing. As you breathe out, bear down on your forearms and fists, and using your toes, hook yourself back a little way.

Variation 5 Still on your stomach, bend your left leg so that your thigh is at an oblique angle to your body, your right leg remaining straight. Bend your right arm and place the palm on the floor a little way in front of you. Bend your left arm as well and place the palm level with your left shoulder. Simultaneously pushing with left foot and pulling with right hand, propel yourself forward. Repeat on the other side. Once you know what you are doing, make left and right part of a single movement instead of two separate movements. And keep it smooth, so that you glide along the floor, exhaling as you move forward.

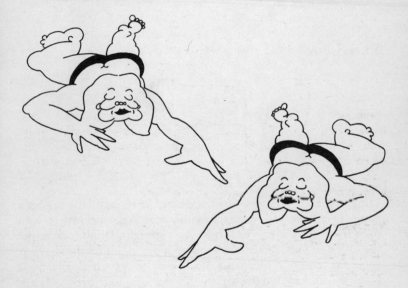

Exercise 5

If you didn't bottom-crawl as a child, now's your chance. Sit on the floor, left leg bent so that the knee skims the floor, right bent but upright. Clasp the right knee with both hands. Bear down on right foot and pull yourself along the floor on your buttocks. Don't get over-enthusiastic, keep it small and concentrate on putting your weight on the right foot. Repeat on the other side.

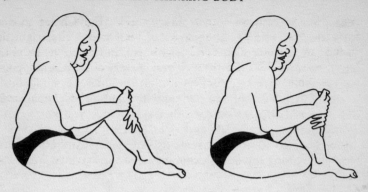

Exercise 6

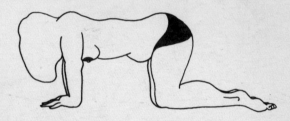

Time to crawl – get on your hands and knees and let your belly hang. In all the following crawling exercises, check that your back has the same curves it has when straight. Don't tuck under the tail, don't straighten the lumbar spine, don't let the thoracic spine sag, and don't let your head hang down. Check that your knees are underneath the hip/thigh joints, not together but apart, though not so far apart as your hands, which should be underneath the arm/shoulder joints – unless, of course, your hips are wider than your shoulders. Check also that your calves are in a straight line with your knees and that your toes are not turned in towards one another. When you crawl, the hands and knees will move in a straight path – one pad, so to speak, directly in line with the one before.

Looking straight ahead, place the left hand one pace forward, followed by the left knee. There is no need to lift your knee high off the ground – just skim it. The right hand moves forward, followed by the right knee. And so on. There is little change in the shape of the back or pelvis as you move your knees forward. To get the hang of it, place a book on your sacrum while you are crawling.

Once you have mastered crawling forwards, crawl backwards and then round in a circle.

Variation 1 This time place left hand forward but followed by the right knee, right hand forward, followed by the left knee and so on. After crawling forwards in this fashion, crawl backwards as well as round in a circle.

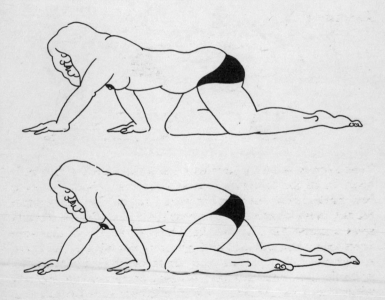

Variation 2   Still in the crawling position, push off from the floor with your hands and, by shifting your calves neatly to the right, sit down to the left of them. Your arms will follow the movement. Rock forwards on to your hands, push back and shift your calves to the left so that you can sit down. Think of it as one continuous movement. If you stop, particularly when you are sitting down, it will be difficult to get up steam to go forward.

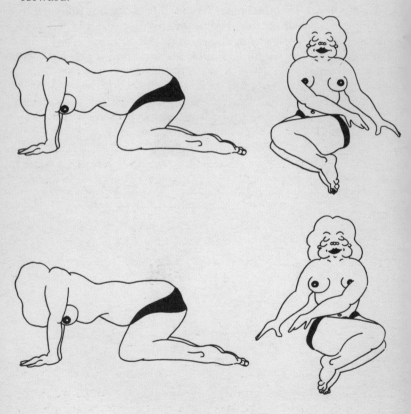

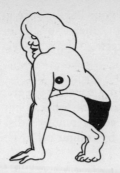

Variation 3   Squat like a rabbit, except that your hands are outside your legs. Move them forward, away from you, and, placing all your weight on them, push forward from the tail as though someone had grabbed you by the seat of your pants; your feet moving up to join your hands. In other words, hop like Peter Rabbit.

Variation 4   Same as above but this time hop backwards. Concentrate on the area at the base of the spine, the sacrum wedged between the two hip bones, spine and tail bone.

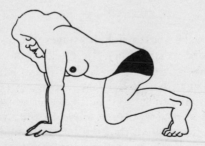

Exercise 7

On all fours for the last time – breathe in, and round the spine, lowering your head and curving your tail bone as though you wanted the two to meet. Make the movement slow and smooth and don't strain. Breathe in as you arch, raising your head and sticking out your bottom as though your tail bone was on a journey to the back of your head. Once again, make the movement slow and smooth; there should be no effort attached. Repeat. This is an exercise to do whenever your back feels as if it needs oiling.

We end as we began – lying on the back, the trunk a pillow full of water, being gently rolled from side to side.

Come to rest on your back, knees bent, arms loosely folded over your chest, and count ten breaths. Come up to sitting slowly and, *as always*, by rolling on to your side.

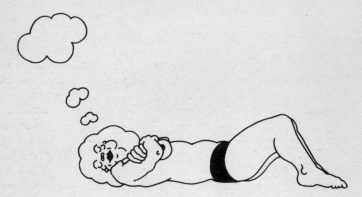

Sitting

The human animal comes upright by stages, the result of a series of moves intended to strengthen the integration of trunk, head and limbs.

Sit on a hard chair with a flat seat. Feel the 'sit bones'; check that your thighs are not splayed out but ever so slightly in, that the calves are set at a 90-degree angle to the thighs, that the feet are flat on the ground, that the heels are under or slightly behind the line of the knee cap, the big toes in a line with the inner edge of the heels.

Focus in on the trunk. Check on the curve of the coccyx, feel the sacrum wedged between the two hip bones, the inner curve of the lumbar spine, the angle of the ribs hanging from the thoracic spine, the brace of the collar bone against the shoulder blades, the balance of the skull on the atlas.

Sitting or standing, the balance of the trunk is no different; the principal change occurs in the relation of the pelvis to the legs. Stand up and check that the pelvis is resting equally on both legs, that the weight of the trunk, head and arms is centred on the hip/thigh sockets. Check that the knuckles of the two thigh bones are resting on both tibias – this will mean that the knees are not locked but feel as if they were slightly bent. Check that the ankle bones are guarding the talus between them, that your weight goes through them and into the heel bones, that it spreads along the outside of the feet to the fifth, fourth and big toes.

To balance all that in the first place, and to maintain that balance in movement, would be much more difficult if the body was an empty container. Too often we think of ourselves in cardboard cut-out fashion, whereas we are three-dimensional and, whatever else their function, our innards are our stabilisers.

Imagine the pelvis as the kind of plastic cylindrical building block you played with as a child. Balance it on a chair and place its contents inside. As you imagine the body made up of building blocks, picture while you're at it what is inside – bowel, colon, kidneys, spleen, liver, stomach, diaphragm, heart, lungs, windpipe, oesophagus, tongue and teeth, hearing tubes, eye-balls and brains, to mention but a few.

Take your load and walk around the room to accustom yourself to the weight. As you walk, check that your feet are turning neither outward nor inward but pointing straight ahead. Slow the movement right down so that you can take in the mechanics. As the heel of the right foot strikes the floor, the left heel leaves the floor (not the foot, just the heel). Your weight is transferred to the right, spreading from the heel along the outside of the right foot to little toes and big toe, and simultaneously the left knee is bringing the left leg forward for the process to be repeated. Speed up your walking, making sure that your pelvis doesn't sag each time the weight is transferred. Check that as the weight is transferred you feel this in the hip/thigh sockets, the trunk balanced atop the pelvis. Brace the shoulder blades with the collar bone, let the arms hang from their sockets, and look around you to free any tension in your neck.

If Big Ben shuffled off the bindings that attach it to the Palace of Westminster and went walk-about, it would be miraculous. Yet the organisational complexity of human walking leaves us unmoved. Far from being astonished by it, we don't even rate it as a feat, unless we have been injured and have to relearn the process.

Like bulls in china shops, we rush to follow the example of those we think of as professionally fit, hoping that some of their grace, strength or stamina will rub off.

Yet dancers will tell you they are always tired, and athletes have been known to get injured. Obsession has a price and pushing the body to extremes too often over too long a period has to be paid for. The role model offered by the professional is of little use to the non-professional.

If we think about what we want from our bodies, it is surely that they will last the course, that they will not burn out before their time, that our old age will not be a succession of painful hours. Luck may play a part, but ours is by far the bigger role.

Summary

The past is past, we must have done with it and allow the twentieth century to provide us with an update. The body thinks, the mind moves in ways that are no longer so mysterious. We are the first generation to have actual as opposed to hypothetical knowledge about ourselves. The past has not been good to the body, and punishing it is even more senseless today when we can no longer plead ignorance.

● Physical jerks are for jerks; the body deserves better. What we possess is not a crude but a sophisticated instrument which we need to learn how to play not bash.

● To do this, we need to rediscover our bodies, relearn the childish stages that brought us to standing and got us moving. To this practical knowledge we must add the theoretical. It is not enough to feel the rightness of a movement, we, being adults, need to know what we are doing.

• We need to practise not by running an extra mile but by putting that knowledge into daily use – watching ourselves as we wash our hair, walk up the stairs, sit down, get up, walk about; remembering the position of the bones and the placement of the muscles. There is nothing like being caught red-handed to make us change our ways. Going over the mechanics in our heads, mentally rehearsing, will soon make homeless the old bad habits. Until the new is second nature to us, all questions of what kind of exercise are academic.

• We, more than previous generations, need to use our bodies intelligently because modern technology has done away with many of our chores and consequently the need for many of our skills. If we are not to degenerate, we need to stop taking our bodies for granted – before they become part of this century's obsolescence.

Glossary

Articulate   form a joint
Articulation   joint
Condyle   knuckle
Facet   joint surface
Foramen (pl. *foramina*)   hole, opening
Fossa   depression
process   roughened projection
Trochanter   process intended as a grip for a muscle
Tubercle   small round process
Tuberosity   large round process

Notes

Chapter 1

1. 'Neurology and the mind-brain problem' (*American Scientist* no. 40, 1952).
2. Wedberg, A., *A History of Philosophy*, vol. 1: Antiquity & the Middle Ages' (Oxford, 1982).
3. Plato, *Timaeus & Critias* (Penguin Classics). This is taken from Timaeus 12: 'The human body: head and limbs'.
4. ibid. 38: 'The mortal parts of the soul'.
5. Bacon, Francis, *Advancement of Learning*.
6. Augustine, St, *The City of God*, book 14, chapter 5.
7. ibid.
8. Plato, *Timaeus & Critias*. Timaeus 46: 'The balance of mind and body'.
9. Descartes, *Discourse on Method and the Meditations*, 6th Meditation (trans. E. V. Rieu).
10. ibid.
11. Sperry, Roger, 'Neurology and the mind-brain problem' (*American Scientist* no. 40, 1952).
12. Ornstein, Robert, *The Psychology of Consciousness*.
13. Koestler, Arthur, *The Sleepwalkers*.
14. ibid.
15. Ornstein, Robert, *Multimind* (Macmillan, 1986).
16. Luria, A. R. [quoting Pavlov], *Higher Cortical Functions in Man* (Basic Books, N. Y., 1980).
17. Sperry, Roger, 'The great cerebral commissure' (*Scientific American* no. 44-52, 1964).

18. Gazzaniga, Michael S., 'The split brain in man' (*Scientific American* no. 24-29, 1967).
19. Semmes, Josephine, 'Hemispheric Specialization: A possible clue to mechanism' (*Neuropsychologia* no. 6, 1968).
20. Geschwind, Norman, and Galaburda, Albert, *Cerebral Lateralization: Biological Mechanisms, Associations and Pathology* (M. I. T. Press, 1987).
21. Luria, A. R. [quoting Pavlov], *Higher Cortical Functions in Man* (Basic Books. N.Y., 1980).
22. ibid.
23. Sperry, Roger, 'Neurology and the mind-brain problem' (*American Scientist* no. 40, 1952).
24. Koestler, Arthur, *The Sleepwalkers.*

Chapter 2

McMinn & Hutchings, *A Colour Atlas of Human Anatomy* (Wolfe Medical Books, London, 1984).
Sweigard, Lulu E., *Human Movement Potential* (Harper & Row, N.Y., 1974).
Duchenne, G. B., *Physiology of Motion* (W. B. Saunders, Philadelphia, 1959).
Todd, Mabel Elsworth, *The Thinking Body* (Dance Horizons Inc., Brooklyn, N.Y.).

Chapter 3

Ornstein, R., Thompson, R. and Macaulay, D., *The Amazing Brain* (Houghton Mifflin, Boston, 1984).
Dekker, Marcel, *Handbook of the Spinal Cord*, N.Y., 1984.
Basmajian, J. V., and de Luca, C. J., *Muscles Alive* (Williams & Wilkins, Baltimore, 1985).
Campbell, E. J. M., and Howell, H. B. L., 'Proprioceptive control of breathing' in Renck, A. V. S., and O'Connor, M. (eds.), *CIBA Foundation Symposium on Pulmonary Structure & Function* (J. & A. Churchill, 1962).

Rankin, J., and Dempsey, J. A., 'Respiratory Muscles and the Mechanisms of Breathing' (*Amercian Journal of Physical Medicine*, vol. 46, no. 1., 1967).

Campbell, E. J. M., Agostini E., and Newsom-Davis, J., *The Respiratory Muscles – Mechanics & Neural Control* (Lloyd-Luke Medical Books, London, 1958).

Flint, M. M. 'Abdominal muscle involvement during the performance of various forms of sit-up exercise' (*American Journal of Physical Medicine*, vol. 44, no. 5, 1965).

Sokoloff, L., and Bland, J. H., *Musculoskeletal System – Structure & Function in Disease* (Williams & Wilkins, Baltimore, 1975).

Keynes, R. D., and Aidley, D. J., *Nerve & Muscle* (Cambridge University Press, 1985).

Chapter 4

Connolly, K. J., 'Child Development – Learning & the concept of critical periods in infancy' (*Developmental Medicine & Child Neurology*, vol. 14, 1972).

Connolly, K. J., 'The nature of motor skill development' (*Journal of Human Movement Studies* vol. 3, 1977).

Bower, T. G. R., *Primer of Infant Development* (W. H. Freeman & Co., San Francisco, 1977).

Mills, M., and Bainbridge Cohen, B., *Developmental Movement Therapy* (Distributed by The Association for Dance Movement Therapy, 99 South Hill Park, London).

Pearce, J. C., *Magical Child* (Bantam Books, 1986).